OXFORD MEDICAL PUBLICATIONS

Coronary Heart Disease

THE FACTS

ALSO PUBLISHED BY OXFORD
UNIVERSITY PRESS

Ageing: the facts
Nicholas Coni, William Davison, and
Stephen Webster

Allergy: the facts
R. Davies and S. Ollier

**Arthritis and rheumatism:
the facts**
J. T. Scott

Asthma: the facts (second edition)
Donald J. Lane and Anthony Storr

Back pain: the facts
(second edition)
Malcolm Jayson

Blood disorders: the facts
Sheila T. Callender

Breast cancer: the facts
(second edition) Michael Baum

Cancer: the facts
Sir Ronald Bodley Scott

Childhood diabetes: the facts
J. O. Craig

Contraception: the facts
(second edition)
Peter Bromwich and Tony Parsons

Cystic fibrosis: the facts
(second edition)
Ann Harris and Maurice Super

Deafness: the facts
Andrew P. Freeland

Down syndrome: the facts
M. Selikowitz

Eating disorders: the facts
(second edition)
S. Abraham and D. Llewellyn-Jones

Epilepsy: the facts
Anthony Hopkins

Head injury: the facts
D. Gronwall, P. Wrightson, and
P. Waddell

Hypothermia: the facts
K. J. Collins

Kidney disease: the facts
(second edition) Stewart Cameron

**Liver disease and gallstones:
the facts**
A. G. Johnson and D. Triger

Migraine: the facts
F. Clifford Rose and M. Gawel

Miscarriage: the facts
G. C. L. Lachelin

Multiple sclerosis: the facts
(second edition) Bryan Matthews

Parkinson's disease: the facts
(second edition)
Gerald Stern and Andrew Lees

Rabies: the facts
(second edition) Colin Kaplan,
G. S. Turner, and D. A. Warrell

**Sexually transmitted diseases:
the facts**
David Barlow

Stroke: the facts
F. Clifford Rose and R. Capildeo

Thyroid disease: the facts
(second edition) R. I. S. Bayliss and
W. M. G. Tunbridge

Coronary Heart Disease

THE FACTS

DESMOND JULIAN

and

CLAIRE MARLEY

Oxford New York Tokyo
OXFORD UNIVERSITY PRESS
1991

Oxford University Press, Walton Street, Oxford OX2 6DP

Oxford New York Toronto
Delhi Bombay Calcutta Madras Karachi
Petaling Jaya Singapore Hong Kong Tokyo
Nairobi Dar es Salaam Cape Town
Melbourne Auckland

and associated companies in
Berlin Ibadan

Oxford is a trade mark of Oxford University Press

Published in the United States
by Oxford University Press, New York

British Library Cataloguing in Publication Data
A catalogue record for this book is
available from the British Library.

Library of Congress Cataloging in Publication Data
Julian, Desmond G. (Desmond Gareth)
Coronary heart disease : the facts / Desmond Julian, Claire Marley
(Oxford medical publications)
1st edn—Coronary heart disease / J.P. Shillingford. 1981.
Includes index.
1. Coronary heart disease—Popular works. I. Julian, Desmond. II. Marley, Claire.
Coronary heart disease. III. Title. IV. Series.
[DNLM: 1. Coronary Disease-popular works. WG 113 J94c]
RC685.C6S5 1991 616.1´23-dc20 90-14368
ISBN 0-19-261934-9 (hbk.)
ISBN 0-19-262016-9 (pbk.)

Typeset by Downdell Ltd, Oxford
Printed in Great Britain
by Biddles Ltd, Guildford & King's Lynn

Preface

Romantic though it may be to consider the heart the seat of our emotions or, looked at more spiritually, as inextricably linked with our 'soul', in reality, the heart is a very well designed and remarkably reliable piece of plumbing.

Most of us take for granted the reliability of that plumbing, subjecting it to repeated tests, assuming it will always surmount the insurmountable. Many of us forget about the strains we put upon our hearts and are even unaware of the hidden risks within our own lifestyles, only being alerted to them once problems have set in.

Sadly, things can and do go wrong all too frequently, with heart attacks affecting over a quarter of a million people in the UK each year and angina over two million. Coronary disease is the biggest killer in the Western world and, although we may wish to console ourselves that heart attacks provide a 'nice way to go' for very elderly people, the truth is that many people—both men and women—die or become ill in the prime of their lives.

We may have read about the 'coronary epidemic' in our newspapers and magazines, but seldom does the truth hit home until it is just that—very close to home. Once faced with a diagnosis as serious as angina or a heart attack, many patients, partners, and relatives are deafened by the thunder of anxiety and fail to hear the advice and information which follows. Others are simply afraid to ask. And haven't we all told ourselves that the doctor is too busy to answer our questions? But there are a lot of questions: Why me? Where did I go wrong? Will I need an operation? Am I going to die? This small book should help to answer some of the unspoken questions, to explain what goes wrong with the heart in coronary disease, what investigations, treatments, and long-term follow-up might be necessary and, perhaps most importantly, the steps we can all take towards preventing such problems recurring or, indeed, happening in the first place.

We hope that anyone interested in their own health or in that of a loved one who is at risk or already a 'heart patient' will find straightforward facts and explanations (enhanced by a Glossary of more technical terms), a greater understanding of the difficulties that may be encountered, and reassurance without platitudes.

London   D.J.
March 1991   C.M.

Contents

1. The heart and the circulation of the blood

The heart is a simple but remarkable pump. It can be relied upon to beat about 60 times a minute for a lifetime without needing maintenance. Its purpose is to deliver blood to the tissues and organs of the body so that they are supplied with all the nutrition and oxygen that they need. It also has to receive the blood returning to it from the body, and pump this through the lungs, where oxygen is picked up and carbon dioxide released.

THE STRUCTURE OF THE HEART

The heart has four chambers—two atria and two ventricles (Fig. 1.1). The blood returning from the body through the veins to the heart first enters the right atrium (from the Latin word for the central courtyard of a Roman house). From there, blood flows into the right ventricle (from the Latin for belly or stomach). It is then pumped out into the pulmonary arteries and through the fine capillary vessels in the lungs, where it gives up carbon dioxide and absorbs oxygen from the incoming air. The blood returns from the lungs to the left atrium and then into the left ventricle, which pumps it out into the aorta, the main blood vessel. The left ventricle has a thick muscular wall which allows it to push blood through the arteries at the high pressure needed to force it through the innumerable small arteries and capillaries in all parts of the body. The job of the right ventricle is less demanding, the pressure required to propel blood through the lungs being much less; its wall is correspondingly thinner. The muscular walls of the two atria, which act more as receiving chambers than pumps, are thinner still.

The heart is mainly composed of muscle, but it is lined on the inside by a thin layer of cells, called the endocardium, and on the outside by a membrane called the pericardium, which forms a double layered sac that encloses the heart. Within the heart there are four valves which ensure that blood flows in only one direction (Fig. 1.1).

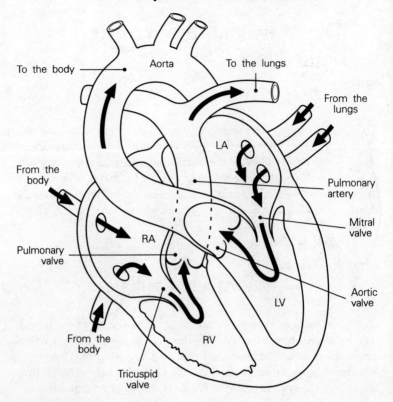

Fig. 1.1. Cross-section of the heart chambers, showing the direction of blood flow and the four valves that ensure that the blood flows in only one direction. (RA = right atrium; LA = left atrium; RV = right ventricle; LV = left ventricle.)

THE CORONARY ARTERIES—THE HEART'S OWN BLOOD SUPPLY

The heart muscle requires its own blood supply and this is provided by the coronary arteries (Fig. 1.2). The right and left main coronary arteries arise from the aorta a short way above the aortic valve, the left soon dividing into two large branches—the anterior descending and the circumflex. Because of this, it is customary to refer to there being three coronary arteries. These large arteries run over the surface of the heart, dividing into smaller branches that plunge through the muscle of the heart as far as the endocardium. These further divide into even smaller arteries and capillaries, whence the blood flows into veins which re-enter the cavity of the heart in the right atrium.

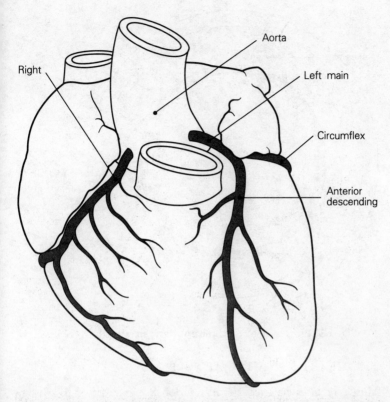

Fig. 1.2. The coronary arteries arising from the aorta, branching and spreading out over the surface of the heart.

The walls of the coronary arteries have three layers (Fig. 1.3):

- An inner lining or 'intima', which consists of a single layer of cells.
- A middle layer or 'media', which is composed of muscle.
- An outer layer or 'adventitia', which is composed of fibres.

The inner and middle layers are separated from each other by a sheet ('lamina') of elastic tissue. The muscle in the walls of the arteries normally controls the amount of blood flowing through them. The muscles are usually slightly contracted, i.e. they have 'tone', which varies constantly as the demand for coronary blood flow changes.

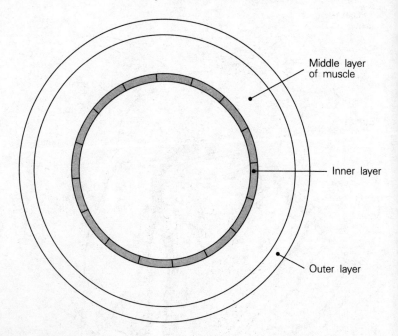

Fig. 1.3. Cross-section of a coronary artery, showing the three layers.

THE HEART'S ELECTRICAL SUPPLY

Muscle requires electrical stimulation for it to contract or 'beat'. The heart generates its own electricity in specialized cells called 'pacemaker' cells (Fig. 1.4). These are located in various parts of the heart, but the most important concentration is in the sinus node, situated in the wall of the right atrium. The sinus node fires off spontaneously, but is under the control of nerves that determine the rate at which it does so. The electrical impulse spreads out over the two atria, but can only reach the ventricles through a slender band of fibres called the 'bundle of His'. Having traversed this, the current spreads out over the two ventricles.

    This orderly sequence of electrical activity leads to a corresponding sequence of contractions (heart beats), so that the atria contract first, and the ventricles shortly thereafter.

    An electrocardiogram (ECG) is a recording of the electrical events occurring in the heart (Fig. 1.5), obtained from signals picked up by electrodes attached to the skin at various sites on the chest and limbs. The first wave (the P wave) represents the atrial current, and the next major wave (called the QRS because it usually has three components)

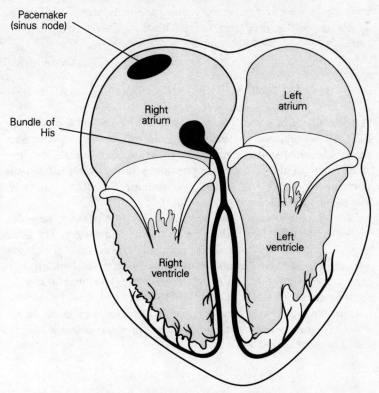

Pacemaker
(sinus node)

Right
atrium

Left
atrium

Bundle of
His

Left
ventricle

Right
ventricle

Fig. 1.4. Electrical pathways of the heart.

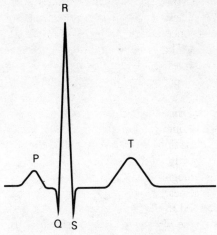

R

P

T

Q S

Fig. 1.5. The normal electrocardiogram.

corresponds to activation of the ventricles. Finally, there is a T wave, which denotes flow of current that restores the ventricles to their resting state.

BLOOD PRESSURE—THE DRIVING FORCE

A certain level of pressure is necessary to drive the blood around the body. Blood pressure is usually measured with a mercury sphygmo-manometer and the measurements are therefore expressed in millimetres of mercury (mmHg). The blood pressure is higher when the heart is pumping ('systole') than when it is relaxing ('diastole'), and both systolic and diastolic pressures are noted.

What is normal varies very much with age (the pressure becoming higher as one gets older), but also with activity and anxiety. The blood pressure is customarily regarded as normal if the systolic is at or below 140 mmHg and the diastolic at or below 90 mmHg (140/90). It is regarded as being high if the systolic is above 160 mmHg and the diastolic above 95 mmHg (160/95). However, a visit to the doctor's surgery can cause anxiety and temporarily increase the pressure; no one should be regarded as having a high blood pressure unless it remains raised on several occasions.

2. What is coronary disease?

The term 'coronary *heart* disease'—or coronary disease for short—is used to describe a disorder of the heart muscle resulting from narrowing of the coronary arteries (see Chapter 1) (i.e. 'coronary *artery* disease'). Because of the narrowing, the heart muscle may not receive sufficient blood: an inadequate blood supply is called 'ischaemia'; the term 'ischaemic heart disease' is synonymous with coronary heart disease. Often the blood supply is only insufficient when demands on the heart are increased as on exercise. This transient ischaemia may cause a chest discomfort called 'angina', which characteristically disappears on rest. When the reduction in blood supply is so severe as to cause death of the muscle cells beyond the obstruction, this is known as 'myocardial infarction', 'myocardial' referring to the heart muscle and 'infarction' to the death of cells. This is often also called a 'coronary' or heart attack.

ATHEROMA AND ATHEROSCLEROSIS

In the vast majority of cases, coronary disease is the result of a process known as atheroma or atherosclerosis. Atheroma refers to soft, fatty material that accumulates in the arteries and is derived from the Greek word for gruel. It usually does so in localized deposits called 'plaques'. The term 'sclerosis' is used to describe the hardening process that may take place as a result of the deposition of fibrous material or calcium (calcification), and is a Greek word for hardness.

WHY DOES ATHEROMA OCCUR?

Atheroma is a result of interactions between the walls of the coronary arteries and the constituents of the blood; these include the blood cells, the clotting factors, and the fats transported in the blood.

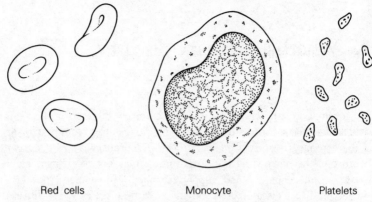

| Red cells | Monocyte | Platelets |

Fig. 2.1. Cells of the blood.

The blood cells (Fig. 2.1)

The red cells are the most numerous and are responsible for carrying oxygen to the tissues of the body. They play no part in the development of coronary disease, but if there are too few of them, as in anaemia, a lack of oxygen may impair the action of the heart muscle.

Most white cells are concerned with defence against infection and injury, and are not involved in the formation of atheroma. However, one type, the monocyte, plays a crucial role when it migrates from the blood into the wall of the artery and provokes changes in the artery.

Platelets are blood cells that stick to the surface of injured blood vessels and have an essential role in stopping bleeding. However, when they form on the surface of a damaged, narrowed artery they clump together to form a clot ('thrombus'). In turn this may trigger off the deposition of a fibrin clot. The clot may become incorporated into the arterial wall and increase the narrowing.

Blood clotting (Fig. 2.2)

The fluid plasma in which the cells of the blood float contains proteins that solidify to form clots. Clotting is an extremely complex process which is of profound importance both in the preservation of the body from injury and in the progression of coronary disease.

The soluble protein *fibrinogen* is a normal constituent of the plasma. It is converted to insoluble *fibrin* to form a clot by an enzyme called *thrombin*. Thrombin is not normally present in the blood (or it would clot), but is produced in response to injury from a substance in the blood, *prothrombin*.

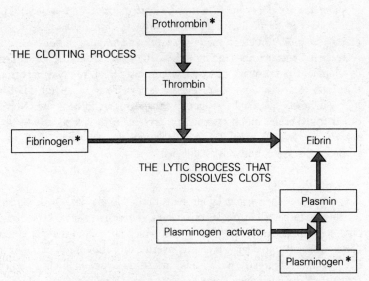

* These inactive substances are normally present in blood but are converted into the active substances, as indicated by the arrows, when there is an injury leading to the process of clotting.

Fig. 2.2. Mechanisms of blood clotting and lysis.

When the inner lining of a coronary artery is damaged, platelets adhere to the site of injury. If the injury is severe enough, this triggers the formation of a fibrin clot.

The dissolving ('lysis') of clots

Fibrin clots can be dissolved (lysed) by *plasmin*. This is not normally active in blood, but is formed from *plasminogen* when the enzyme *plasminogen activator* acts on it, as it does in the presence of clot. Plasminogen activator is a naturally occurring substance, but there are a number of 'thrombolytic' or 'fibrinolytic' drugs available that simulate its action (see Chapter 6).

Fats in the blood

Various fatty substances in the blood are related to the development of coronary disease. The best known of these is cholesterol which when bound to proteins becomes what is known as a *lipoprotein*. Depending upon which type of protein the cholesterol is bound to, it may form part of a *low density lipoprotein* (LDL) or a *high density lipoprotein* (HDL). LDL has been particularly linked to coronary disease, because it is a major component of atheromatous plaques and because there is a strong relationship between the amount of LDL in the blood and the subsequent development of coronary disease. By contrast, HDL removes fats from the walls of arteries; coronary disease is less likely when the HDL is high—it has been called the 'good' cholesterol. Another type of fat is called triglyceride, much of which is present in the blood as *very low density lipoprotein* (VLDL). The relationship between VLDL and coronary disease is not well established.

Fats in the diet

The amount of the various lipoproteins in the blood is largely dependent on the fat rather than cholesterol eaten. There is usually little actual cholesterol in the diet, and most of that which appears in the circulation comes from saturated fat, which is converted into cholesterol in the liver. Fats (or more correctly fatty acids) in the diet vary in their chemical structure. The fats contain a chain of carbon atoms joined to each other by bonds. Each carbon atom has four bonds which can link it to other atoms; two usually form the link with the adjacent carbon atoms and the remaining two are 'saturated' with hydrogen (H) atoms (Fig. 2.3). If not all carbon bonds are saturated in this way, they can form a double link with an adjacent carbon atom and are then said to be 'unsaturated'. If there is one such double bond present, as in the oleic acid of olive oil, the fat is said to be 'monounsaturated'; if there is more than one, as in the linoleic acid of sunflower oil, it is said to be 'polyunsaturated'. Saturated fats tend to increase the level of LDL, whereas the unsaturated oils tend to lower it.

THE FORMATION OF ATHEROMA

As described in Chapter 1, the walls of the coronary arteries are composed of three layers. The inner layer, which is in direct contact with the blood, consists of a single sheet of cells. The middle layer is mainly made up of muscle cells, and the outer layer of fibres.

A common finding in all parts of the world is that streaks of fat occur in the inner layer of the coronary arteries, but it is only in communities that have a high incidence of coronary disease that these are liable to progress to something more sinister—the development of substantial deposits or plaques (Fig. 2.4). Several factors (as outlined above) seem to contribute to these—the behaviour of platelets and monocytes, an invasion of muscle cells from the middle layer, and the infiltration of fat and cholesterol from the blood. These plaques tend to form in the larger

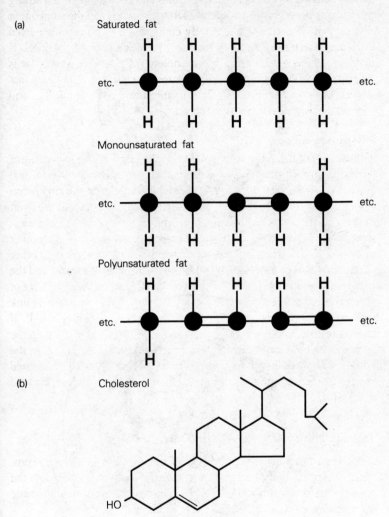

Fig. 2.3. Chemical structure of (a) fats and (b) cholesterol. Note that there are only single bonds joining carbon atoms (black circles) in saturated fats, while there is one double bond in monounsaturated fats, and two or more in poly-unsaturated fats.

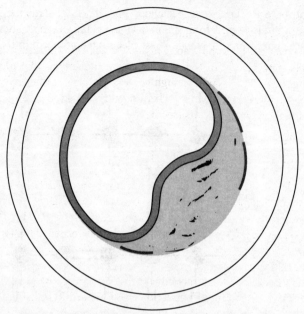

Fig. 2.4. Plaque formation narrowing a coronary artery.

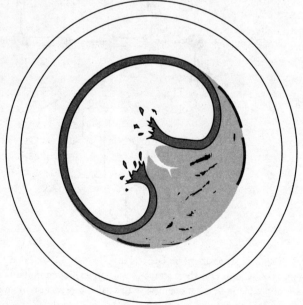

Fig. 2.5. Plaque rupture, the cap over a plaque fissuring—often the first event in
a heart attack.

arteries, and in due course they narrow the artery so much that insufficient blood may reach the muscle beyond. The plaque is separated from the bloodstream by a thin cap. This may crack (Fig. 2.5); if it does so, platelets may adhere to the site of injury, and initiate the process of clotting. If the clot is large enough to block the artery, the heart muscle cells beyond the obstruction may be so severely deprived of oxygen that a myocardial infarction results (see below).

OTHER INFLUENCES ON THE BLOOD SUPPLY TO HEART MUSCLE

Two additional factors influence the blood supply of the heart muscle—the state of contraction (tone) of the muscle in the walls of the coronary arteries and the presence or absence of collateral vessels.

Blood flow in the coronary arteries is largely determined by the degree of contraction or relaxation of the muscular walls of the small coronary arteries that run deep in the muscle of the heart. These relax when more blood is required and contract when the need lessens. Most of the time they are in a state of mild contraction that is described as having 'tone'. Normally, increases in tone in the larger arteries have little effect on blood flow, but if the arteries are severely narrowed by atheroma, they may cause ischaemia.

Occasionally, an artery which is otherwise free of disease suddenly becomes severely narrowed by 'spasm' (see also Chapter 7). This rare condition usually occurs in episodes of angina lasting a few minutes at a time, which tend to be unassociated with exercise and are particularly likely in the early morning. The cause of coronary spasm is unknown.

Normally, each artery is solely responsible for an area of heart muscle; therefore, if an artery is suddenly blocked, the muscle beyond the block dies because there is no alternative blood supply. If, however, an artery narrows slowly and progressively, new blood vessels called 'collaterals' develop from adjacent arteries and can provide the threatened territory with enough blood to prevent infarction if complete blockage ensues.

WHAT HAPPENS IN A MYOCARDIAL INFARCTION?

As described above, the first stage of a myocardial infarction is most often a tearing of the cap covering a plaque; this is followed by platelet and then fibrin clotting (Fig. 2.6). Usually, this causes complete obstruction of the artery and the muscle beyond dies, the amount affected

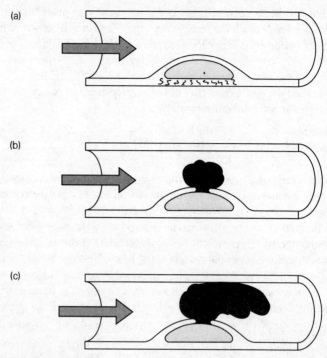

Fig. 2.6. Coronary thrombosis: (a) plaque in a coronary artery wall; (b) plaque rupture and clot formation; (c) blockage. The arrow shows the direction of blood flow.

depending upon the area of muscle supplied by the blocked artery and also upon collateral flow. In many patients, only a small part of the heart is damaged, there are no complications and recovery is excellent. However, it is potentially a serious disorder because of several complications that may arise, as follows.

VENTRICULAR FIBRILLATION—CARDIAC ARREST

The dying muscle may start a rhythm disturbance called 'ventricular fibrillation' in which the electrical activity of the ventricles becomes totally disorganized. The heart cannot pump out any blood, and the condition of cardiac arrest results. This is almost invariably fatal unless it is treated very promptly (see p. 60). Ventricular fibrillation is particularly common in the first hour after the onset of the attack, becoming progressively less frequent over the next six hours. If the patient survives this period, the outcome depends largely upon the extent of muscle damage.

SHOCK AND HEART FAILURE

If as much as 40 per cent of the heart muscle is damaged, there is usually not enough pumping power left to maintain the circulation. The condition known as shock develops in which the blood pressure drops and the patient becomes pale, cold, and sometimes blue, and is mentally confused. Death often follows within the next few hours. With less severe damage, the blood pressure may be preserved but the left ventricle cannot cope with all the blood returning to it from the lungs, and these become congested. The patient becomes breathless and distressed, but medical treatment can usually correct the situation quite quickly.

OTHER COMPLICATIONS

The muscle of the heart may become so weakened that blood may force its way through the wall into the pericardium or through the septum between the two ventricles, causing a 'ventricular septal defect'. Both these forms of 'cardiac rupture' are usually fatal very quickly, but occasionally the defect can be repaired surgically.

When the muscle of the heart dies, it is replaced by fibrous tissue. Sometimes, this becomes very thin; if a large area is involved, this part of the heart may be pushed out as the rest of the muscle is contracting. Such an area is known as an 'aneurysm'. Small aneurysms do not pose much of a problem, but larger ones mean that the remaining heart muscle is wasting much of its energy on useless activity and heart failure may occur. The surgical removal of an aneurysm may restore good function.

Clots tend to form when blood is static. After a heart attack, there are three sites where this may happen:

- in the veins of the legs if bed rest is prolonged;
- in the atria if they are affected by a rhythm disturbance known as atrial fibrillation;
- in the left ventricle adjacent to a large area of dead muscle.

In each case, a clot may break off and migrate to another part of the body, causing an 'embolism'. Clots from the leg veins may go to the lungs, causing obstruction by pulmonary embolism; this was a common cause of death in former days when patients were kept in bed for weeks after a heart attack. Emboli from the left side of the heart are most likely to go to the brain, causing a stroke.

3. Who develops coronary heart disease and why?

Coronary heart disease is now generally recognized as 'the captain of the men of death', just as tuberculosis was 50 years ago. The pre-eminence of coronary disease today is partly due to the almost complete eradication of many infectious diseases, but there has also been a very real increase in heart attacks in most Western countries.

It is difficult to know whether the disease was present in the ancient world. Certainly, atheroma (see Chapter 2) was found when post-mortems were done on Egyptian mummies of 1000 BC and also on Chinese mummies. However, although scholars have tried to identify the symptoms of coronary disease in the illnesses of famous people in the intervening years, there are few convincing examples. It was only in the late eighteenth century that angina pectoris was first described as a distinctive symptom and not until some years later that its cause was recognized to be in the coronary arteries. From then on, many cases of sudden death were attributed to blockage of the coronary arteries, but the idea that a coronary heart attack could be survived did not take hold until 1912 with the publications of Herrick, an eminent American physician. The first cases of myocardial infarction were not diagnosed in British hospitals until the 1920s, and the diagnosis remained rare until the 1930s. It was not until the electrocardiogram (ECG) came into widespread use that non-fatal heart attacks were found to be common. The enormous upsurge in the number of coronary deaths in the United States and Europe after the Second World War, and their subsequent decline in some countries, is a matter of the greatest interest and will be discussed in detail below.

WHO SUFFERS FROM CORONARY DISEASE?

Most of what we know about the causes of coronary disease comes from epidemiological studies, that is, those that have compared the prevalence of the disease in different populations, or observed its development in large groups of carefully studied, apparently normal individuals.

Coronary heart disease is relatively rare in Japan (as it is in mainland China), but it is also not very common in the Mediterranean countries including Spain, Italy (especially the south), and Greece. By contrast the British Isles and Scandinavia have some of the worst records in the world. Even within Britain, there are great variations in the numbers dying of coronary disease. In 1987, in Scotland and Northern Ireland some 480 people out of every 100 000 died of coronary disease, compared with 350 in East Anglia. Men and women from the subcontinent of India living in the United Kingdom are more likely to develop coronary disease than the white population living in the same area.

Men are more likely to die of coronary disease than are women, although the difference becomes progressively less after the menopause. In both sexes, deaths from coronary disease increase with advancing age.

LARGE-SCALE POPULATION STUDIES

Two famous studies—the Seven Countries Study and the Framingham Study (from the United States)—provided much of the basis for the beliefs held today about the risk factors for coronary disease (see also Chapter 4), but they have been amplified by many other studies in a variety of countries. In Britain, important information about the regional differences in deaths from coronary disease has been provided by the Office of Population Censuses and Surveys, the British Regional Heart Study, the Scottish Heart Health Study, and the Caerphilly Study in Wales.

In the Seven Countries Study, groups of men from the United States, Japan, Yugoslavia, Finland, Italy, The Netherlands, and Greece were examined and then followed up for ten years or more. The importance of blood cholesterol as a risk factor was striking (see below), with very few individuals in Japan, Greece, and Yugoslavia having high levels of cholesterol or developing coronary disease, in contrast with Finland and the United States where both were common. The blood cholesterol levels in the different countries correlated well with the proportion of saturated fat in the diet.

In the Framingham Study, some 5000 men and women aged between 30 and 59 years were examined in the late 1940s; many of them have now been followed up for more than 20 years. The chief findings have been the importance of blood cholesterol, cigarette smoking, and high blood pressure. Essentially, all the other studies have reinforced this message, but coronary disease is rare in communities (such as the

Japanese) with low cholesterol levels even if they smoke a lot and have a high incidence of hypertension (high blood pressure).

WHAT ARE THE RISK FACTORS FOR CORONARY DISEASE?

The term 'risk factor' is used to describe a feature that is associated with the development of coronary disease (see also Chapter 4). Strictly speaking one should talk about 'risk associations' unless one is sure that the factor is causal. Thus, a white ring around the cornea at a young age (corneal arcus) is associated with the premature development of coronary disease, but no one would suggest that this is causative, nor would one expect that removing an eye would prevent coronary disease! Similarly, it has been found that in the United Kingdom and the United States, small men are more likely to get coronary disease than tall men—would their risk be reduced by wearing high heels? Curiously, the small Japanese have a low incidence of the disease, but when they migrate to the United States they grow taller and have more coronary disease. Clearly, the smallness observed in Britain is not a risk factor itself but is a marker of something else—possibly poor nutrition in youth.

It is extremely important to recognize that there is no single cause of coronary disease, and that almost all those affected have two or more factors, some of which may not yet have been identified.

CHOLESTEROL, DIETARY FACTORS, AND OVERWEIGHT

The relationship between blood cholesterol level and coronary disease has been demonstrated in many studies. Perhaps the most impressive evidence comes from the Multiple Risk Factor Intervention Trial (known as MR FIT), in which 361 662 men were followed up for six years. As will be seen from Fig. 3.1, the relationship between cholesterol and mortality was strong, being particularly evident at high levels. However, even at a level of 7.2 millimoles per litre (mmol/l), only 1.5 per cent of patients died within the six-year period. Furthermore, the risk of coronary death is present even with the lower levels of cholesterol, 0.5 per cent of men with the 'normal' level of 5.2 mmol/l dying within the same time period. In the MR FIT study, 35 per cent of coronary deaths occurred in the 20 per cent of individuals with highest cholesterols, while 65 per

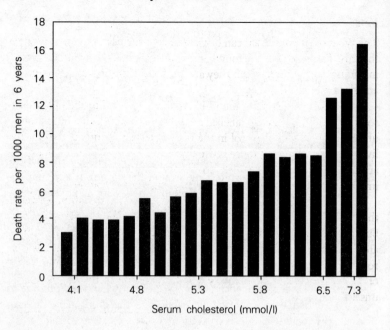

Fig. 3.1. The relationship between the cholesterol level and death rate (from the MR FIT trial).

cent of coronary deaths occurred in those with only slightly raised cholesterol levels. It is the low density component of the cholesterol (LDL) that is most responsible for coronary disease; the high density component (HDL) appears to be protective. The LDL level is partly determined genetically, but it is also largely dependent upon the saturated fat (see p. 10) in the diet; polyunsaturated fat tends to lower it. Whether triglycerides (very low density lipoproteins—VLDL) are risk factors remains controversial—some studies have suggested that they are, but others have not. They would seem to be of little importance unless the blood cholesterol is also raised.

There has been great interest in diet as a factor in coronary disease, partly because of the obvious importance of blood cholesterol levels, and partly because it is probable that the very different incidences of coronary disease in different communities could be, at least partially, explained by differences in food intake. Most attention has focused on the amount and nature of the fats in the diet.

Fats

The types of fat consumed can be classified on the basis of how saturated they are. Saturated fats are found predominantly in food of animal origin, including dairy products, but they are also found in palm oil, coconut oil, and hard margarines.

Polyunsaturated fats are found in sunflower oil and maize oil, and in soft margarines if they are labelled as polyunsaturated. Olive oil is mono-unsaturated. The cholesterol in the body is largely manufactured in the liver from saturated fat; there is usually only a relatively small amount of actual cholesterol in the diet, so dietary cholesterol is of much less importance than saturated fat in causing high blood lipid levels.

In the Seven Countries Study, there was a strong correlation between the incidence of coronary disease and the consumption of saturated fat, but there was an even stronger one with the relative ratio of polyunsaturated and saturated fat consumed (Fig. 3.2). Thus in Japan, there was a roughly equivalent amount of polyunsaturates and saturates eaten (ratio of 1), but in Finland a relatively small proportion of the fat was polyunsaturated.

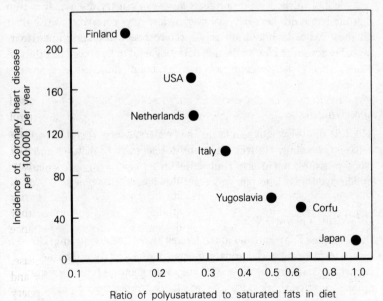

Fig. 3.2. The relationship between the ratio of polyunsaturated to saturated fat in the diet and the incidence of coronary disease in different countries. From Shaper AG, Marr J. Br Med J 1977; 1: 867–71. With permission.

Salt, sugar, and vitamins

Other factors in the diet that have been implicated in coronary disease include salt and sugar. Neither probably plays an important role in this regard. Salt may contribute to high blood pressure in some people and should not be taken in excess.

Sugar contributes to obesity, and may thereby increase both blood pressure and triglycerides; it has no nutritional value other than calories, and is therefore by no means as good a source of carbohydrates as, for example, is fruit.

Vitamins C and E (found in vegetables and fruit) probably protect against the development of coronary disease.

Coffee and alcohol

There have been some reports about coffee being associated with increased coronary disease, and also putting up the cholesterol level. The evidence is not strong and what there is suggests that it is only boiled coffee that is harmful.

There is a widespread belief, based on some epidemiological studies, that alcohol in moderation protects against coronary disease. It is true that moderate drinkers have a lower incidence of coronary disease than do those who do not drink at all or are heavy drinkers, but this is probably accounted for by the fact that they tend to live more healthily in other respects, such as eating a better diet, taking more exercise, and not smoking.

Overweight

The role of overweight as a factor in coronary disease is still a matter of debate. It certainly contributes to the development of diabetes and high blood pressure, but it also contributes in its own right, particularly in middle-aged men who put on weight rapidly and in women.

CIGARETTE SMOKING

In the United Kingdom and in the United States, the relationship between cigarette smoking and coronary disease is very clearly established. It is particularly striking in those who start young and in heavy smokers. In studies on British doctors, the mortality from coronary disease was increased in smokers almost five-fold at 35 to 44 years of age, and nearly four-fold between 45 and 54 years. The differences became less marked with increasing age. In the Framingham Study, in men followed up for

24 years, coronary heart disease was more than twice as common in smokers than in non-smokers for those who were 30 to 39 years old at the start of the study, 1.4 times as common for those between 40 and 49 years, and 1.2 times for those between 50 and 59 years. Heavy smokers in Japan have a higher rate of coronary disease than non-smokers, but have a very much lower incidence of coronary disease than do British men who smoke as much. It would seem that smoking has relatively little effect if the cholesterol is low. Those who smoke cigars or pipes have a lower rate of coronary disease than do cigarette smokers.

HIGH BLOOD PRESSURE

This is the third of the main risk factors. Its relationship to coronary disease has been confirmed in several studies and applies to both the systolic and diastolic levels (see p. 6). Again, in Japan, high blood pressure, which is very common there, is not so strongly associated with coronary disease as it is in the West.

PHYSICAL ACTIVITY

There is impressive evidence that physical exercise, particularly as a leisure activity, protects against the development of coronary disease, but it is curious that perhaps the highest rate of coronary disease in the world is seen in the extremely energetic Finnish lumberjacks. They are, however, heavy smokers and have high cholesterol levels.

A warning is necessary with regard to very vigorous exercise in middle-aged people who are out of training. Probably worst of all in this respect is squash, in which the competitive element is so strong that players may ignore any symptoms they experience in order to win.

DIABETES MELLITUS

There is a considerably increased incidence of coronary disease in patients with diabetes. The reason for this is not certain. It seems that the disease may affect the heart and blood vessels in other ways as well, but the high fat, low carbohydrate diets that used to be given to diabetics might be a factor.

GOUT

Coronary disease is relatively common in sufferers from gout but it is not clear why this is so.

STRESS AND PERSONALITY

There is a widespread popular belief that stress is the main cause of coronary disease. The media image of the coronary patient is that of a high-powered executive, living on his nerves and wedded to his portable telephone. What has become apparent in recent years is that if there is an archetypal coronary patient it is the labourer in the Glasgow docks. Doctors used to have a high incidence of coronary disease and it was then not surprising that they attributed their susceptibility to the stress of their jobs. Heart attacks are now below average amongst doctors but it is unlikely that their stress has become less; the change is most likely due to their reduced consumption of cigarettes. Those who believe that stress is an important factor in coronary disease are now more likely to attribute this to the strain of working under pressure at a repetitive job with little control over the workload. There is still a lot to be learned about what role, if any, stress has as a risk factor; unfortunately it is the most difficult risk factor to quantify.

Two doctors from San Francisco, Friedman and Rosenman, described a 'type A' personality which they considered at high risk of coronary disease. The type A person is highly competitive, and is obsessed with achieving an unlimited number of things in the shortest possible time. His body movements are rapid, and he is inclined to explosive speech, taut facial gestures, and excessive hand movements. These features are perhaps typical of the American executive but do not seem characteristic of the average labourer, who is much more likely to have coronary disease. Some observers from other countries have reported findings similar to those of Friedman and Rosenman, whereas others have not. It seems quite probable that certain psychological characteristics are associated with coronary disease, but they may not be quite as distinctive as Friedman and Rosenman proposed. Some of the more convincing studies have suggested that hostility and suppressed anger may be strongly associated with coronary disease; one could readily see how such emotions would generate the release of the 'fight or flight' hormone adrenaline, which might be harmful.

SOCIAL CLASS

Contrary to what is widely believed, death from coronary heart disease is substantially higher in manual workers than in non-manual workers in the United Kingdom. This can be partly, but not wholly, accounted for by the higher rates of smoking, higher blood pressures, and less leisure-time physical activity in the manual groups.

SEX HORMONES

Coronary disease is rare in menstruating women, but becomes increasingly common after the menopause. Oral contraceptives, particularly high-dose oestrogen pills, have been associated with an increase in coronary disease, but this is largely confined to women over 35 years who smoke, or who have a high cholesterol. Men given oestrogens for the treatment of cancer of the prostate also seem to have an increased risk of coronary disease. By contrast, there is evidence that hormone replacement therapy with oestrogens reduces the risk in post-menopausal women. It is less certain whether the now commonly used combined pill (with progestogen) is also protective.

FAMILY HISTORY

Coronary disease is often suffered by several members of a family; this is particularly likely to be the case when coronary disease occurs at a young age. In some families, there is a clear-cut, inherited abnormality. The best known example of this is familial hyperlipidaemia (high blood fats), in which it has been shown that there is a specific abnormality in the genes. In these cases, there is a defect in the way the liver handles cholesterol, as a result of which the blood cholesterol is extremely high. There are other types of inherited disorders of fat, possibly 1 to 2 per cent of the population being affected in this way. Minor genetic abnormalities may also contribute to high cholesterol levels in a much higher percentage, but the occurrence of coronary disease in families may also be due to a shared environment—for example, members of the same family may smoke heavily or eat the same fatty diet.

WHY HAVE THERE BEEN SUCH IMMENSE CHANGES IN THE DEATHS FROM CORONARY DISEASE IN DIFFERENT COUNTRIES?

In the 1940s and 1950s, there was a remarkable increase in the number of deaths from coronary disease in the United States and Australia. Starting in the 1960s, there has been an equally remarkable decline, so that the present mortality rate is less than half of what it was in 1968. The fall in England and Wales is much less striking—about 12 per cent —so that while the American deaths were 30 per cent more in 1968,

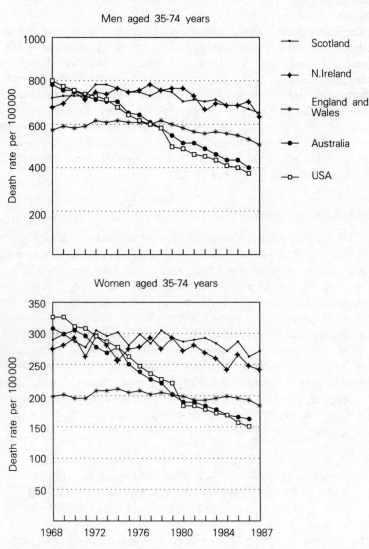

Fig. 3.3. Changing death rates from coronary heart disease among men and women in different countries.

they are now some 25 per cent less (Fig. 3.3). Major falls have also occurred in Canada, the Netherlands, Belgium, and New Zealand.

The reasons for these swings are far from clear. The most obvious change in most of the countries concerned has been a reduction in cigarette smoking. In the United States, there has been only a minor reduction in fat consumption, but a great increase in the proportion taken as polyunsaturated fat. Better care of patients with coronary disease (such as coronary surgery and the development of coronary care units) may also have contributed, but the reduction of deaths is much greater than could be explained by medical treatment alone.

4. The prevention of coronary disease

There is, as yet, no absolute proof that any known measures prevent coronary disease but the differences between countries (see Chapter 3), the changes that have taken place within them, and the changes in incidence that are seen when populations move from one area to another all suggest that there are environmental influences which, if controlled, could reduce the risk of a heart attack and angina. It therefore seems prudent to correct the risk factors (Chapter 3) that have been implicated in coronary disease.

THE CORRECTION OF RISK FACTORS

Table 4.1. Coronary disease risk factors

Established

Raised blood cholesterol level
Diet rich in saturated fat
Cigarette smoking
High blood pressure
Family history of coronary disease at an early age
Gender
Diabetes mellitus

Less well established

Overweight
Lack of physical activity
Socio-economic status
Stress
Oral contraception
Medical conditions such as gout

DIET AND CHOLESTEROL

High levels of blood cholesterol—especially in the form of low density lipoproteins—are clearly related to the incidence of coronary disease; it seems logical that a reduction in blood cholesterol would be effective in reducing the risk.

Most people in Britain have blood cholesterol levels much in excess of the 5.2 mmol/l (millimoles per litre) now generally recommended as the upper limit of normal. It seems sensible, therefore, that virtually everyone should adhere to a diet that keeps their cholesterol low. This applies particularly to young people who have not yet become habituated to a high level, but it is probably never too late to start on such a diet.

Regrettably, doctors have argued with each other for years as to whether lowering cholesterol by diet (or any other means) is desirable. One reason for their scepticism is that many of them demand proof that lowering cholesterol is beneficial. Unfortunately, it is virtually impossible to prove that changes in diet over many years lead to a reduction in the risk of heart attacks. Thus, it is not practicable to assign randomly one group of young people to a low fat diet and another group to a high fat diet and expect them to adhere to it for 10 to 20 years, while doctors wait to see what happens. It is therefore highly improbable that the effectiveness of dietary measures will ever be adequately tested.

Can lowering cholesterol be harmful?

It has been suggested that it might be harmful to lower blood cholesterol, particularly in those who have lived with a high level for many years. It is true that there is some evidence that those with low cholesterols have a higher risk of cancer. This is partly explained by the fact that cancer may lower cholesterol; in this case the cancer is the cause of the low cholesterol and not the other way round. This may not be the whole explanation for the relationship, and anxiety on this score was enhanced by the study of one lipid-lowering agent (clofibrate) that seemed, in a controlled trial, to increase the risk of cancer. It has also been suggested that there is a higher incidence of violent death in those receiving lipid-lowering treatment, but this too is unproven. In spite of these concerns, the benefits of lowering cholesterol appear to outweigh substantially the risks of doing so.

What should we do?

Cutting down on saturated fat

Take only very occasionally:
  Fatty meats, e.g. liver, kidneys, heart, duck, goose, bacon, sausages and other meat products
  Lard, suet, butter, full fat milk, cream, fatty cheeses (e.g. cheddar), cakes, biscuits and chocolate
  Palm oil, coconut oil, hydrogenated vegetable oils

Take in moderation (e.g. 2–3 times a week):
  Lean beef, pork and lamb, less fatty cheeses (e.g. Brie, Edam), eggs

This leaves many excellent and delicious foods of which you can eat as much as you like—chicken and turkey (though not the skin), veal, fish, game (e.g. venison, rabbit), egg whites, virtually all vegetables and fruit, pasta, bread (preferably wholemeal), rice, cereals and oats, olive oil, oils labelled 'polyunsaturated'

NB. There are now many cookbooks that cater for the health-conscious gourmet (see Appendix C)

In 1984, the Committee on Medical Aspects of Food Policy (COMA) produced recommendations on diet which have been widely supported. These were that fat should provide no more than 35 per cent of the calories one eats (compared with an average of some 42 per cent in Britain at the time). The Committee further recommended that not more than 15 per cent of energy should come from saturated fatty acids, and that the ratio of polyunsaturated fatty acids to saturated should be increased.

How can these dietary targets be achieved? By avoiding those foods that contain a large amount of saturated fat and substituting them with fibre and monounsaturated and polyunsaturated fats.

Is fish really good for us?

Fish makes an excellent alternative to meat. White fish is a good source of protein and contains little fat. The fat in fatty fish, such as herring, tuna, salmon, and trout, is predominantly polyunsaturated. Fish oils are

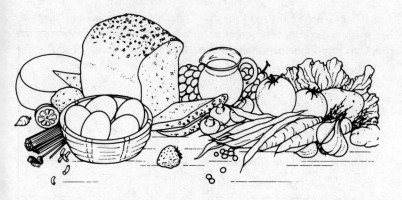

chemically different from other fats and are thought by some to have particularly beneficial effects, although this has yet to be established. It is largely based on the belief that Eskimos, who eat enormous quantities of fatty fish, are relatively free of coronary disease. Whether this is true or not, there is a strong case for increasing fish consumption, and having fatty fish at least twice a week.

What about sugar and salt?

Sugar provides calories but no other value as a food. There is no direct connection between sugar consumption and coronary disease, but as it contributes to obesity and diabetes, and in so far as these are associated with high blood pressure and coronary disease, excessive sugar consumption should be avoided.

There have been alarming stories about the risks of salt, but there is very little evidence that it is a factor in coronary disease. There is more of a connection with high blood pressure but even here the evidence that it plays a causal role is far from established, except in a few people. Certainly, it is unwise for those with heart failure to eat a lot of salt. A prudent approach is to add as little salt as possible in cooking, little or no salt at the table, and to avoid the saltiest foods (for example, crisps; 'convenience foods' such as hamburgers; many processed cold meats).

Fibre

Fibre is a topic that is currently attracting great attention from 'foodies' and food manufacturers. Excessive claims have been made for the cholesterol-lowering potential of some products but there is little doubt that many people eat too little fibre, which is important not only with regard to coronary disease but also in helping to prevent cancer of the bowel. Fruit and vegetables are especially good sources, particularly in the raw state. Wholemeal flour, oats, and pulses are all excellent sources, but there is little proof that one foodstuff is superior to another.

Weight reduction

Overweight is extremely common; everyone should attempt to be within the 'acceptable range' (see Table 4.2). By doing so, one will reduce the risk of high blood pressure, diabetes, and coronary disease. Furthermore, the heart will not have to carry around an unnecessary burden.

The way to a healthy heart

Overweight

Don't get overweight in the first place

If you are above the acceptable range, try to reduce your weight, starting today

Your doctor or a dietician may supply you with a diet sheet

Do not go on a crash diet—do it slowly (about 1 kilo [2 lb] a week)

The only good way to lose weight is to cut down on calories: as fat provides more calories than carbohydrates and protein, the first thing to do is to cut down on fat—especially cakes, sweets, biscuits, crisps, cream, butter, margarine (use a low fat spread instead), and fatty meat—also cut out added sugar; substitute lots of vegetables, salads and high fibre foods

Take more daily exercise

Cooking

At least as important as the food itself is the way in which it is cooked. Preferably food should be grilled, boiled, steamed, or roasted on a rack rather than fried—but if fried, a polyunsaturated oil should be used. Try to eat more raw or lightly cooked vegetables.

Coffee

A small cloud hangs over coffee drinking because boiled coffee appears to raise blood cholesterol, and because in certain studies deaths from

Table 4.2(a)

Men: weight without clothes (st)
(add 6lbs if you weigh yourself in your clothes)

Height	Average weight	Acceptable weight range	Obese
5ft 2in	8st 11lb	8st 0lb–10st 1lb	12st 1lb
5ft 3in	9st 1lb	8st 3lb–10st 4lb	12st 5lb
5ft 4in	9st 4lb	8st 6lb–10st 8lb	12st 10lb
5ft 5in	9st 7lb	8st 9lb–10st 12lb	13st 0lb
5ft 6in	9st 10lb	8st 12lb–11st 2lb	13st 5lb
5ft 7in	10st 0lb	9st 2lb–11st 7lb	13st 11lb
5ft 8in	10st 5lb	9st 6lb–11st 12lb	14st 3lb
5ft 9in	10st 9lb	9st 10lb–12st 2lb	14st 8lb
5ft 10in	10st 13lb	10st 0lb–12st 6lb	14st 13lb
5ft 11in	11st 4lb	10st 4lb–12st 11lb	15st 5lb
6ft 0in	11st 8lb	10st 8lb–13st 2lb	15st 11lb
6ft 1in	11st 12lb	10st 12lb–13st 7lb	16st 3lb
6ft 2in	12st 3lb	11st 2lb–13st 12lb	16st 9lb
6ft 3in	12st 8lb	11st 6lb–14st 3lb	17st 1lb
6ft 4in	12st 13lb	11st 10lb–14st 8lb	17st 7lb

Men: weight without clothes (kg)
(add 3 kg if you weigh yourself in your clothes)

Height	Average weight	Acceptable weight range	Obese
1.60m	57.6kg	52kg–65kg	78kg
1.62m	58.6kg	53kg–66kg	79kg
1.64m	59.6kg	54kg–67kg	80kg
1.66m	60.6kg	55kg–69kg	83kg
1.68m	61.7kg	56kg–71kg	85kg
1.70m	63.5kg	58kg–73kg	88kg
1.72m	65.0kg	59kg–74kg	89kg
1.74m	66.5kg	60kg–75kg	90kg
1.76m	68.0kg	62kg–77kg	92kg
1.78m	69.4kg	64kg–79kg	95kg
1.80m	71.0kg	65kg–80kg	96kg
1.82m	72.6kg	66kg–82kg	98kg
1.84m	74.2kg	67kg–84kg	101kg
1.86m	75.8kg	69kg–86kg	103kg
1.88m	77.6kg	71kg–88kg	106kg

Table 4.2(b)

Women: weight without clothes (st)
(add 4lbs if you weigh yourself in your clothes)

Height	Average weight	Acceptable weight range	Obese
4ft 10in	7st 4lb	6st 8lb– 8st 7lb	10st 3lb
4ft 11in	7st 6lb	6st 10lb– 8st 10lb	10st 6lb
5ft 0in	7st 9lb	6st 12lb– 8st 13lb	10st 10lb
5ft 1in	7st 12lb	7st 1lb– 9st 2lb	11st 0lb
5ft 2in	8st 1lb	7st 4lb– 9st 5lb	11st 3lb
5ft 3in	8st 4lb	7st 7lb– 9st 8lb	11st 7lb
5ft 4in	8st 8lb	7st 10lb– 9st 12lb	11st 12lb
5ft 5in	8st 11lb	7st 13lb–10st 2lb	12st 2lb
5ft 6in	9st 2lb	8st 2lb–10st 6lb	12st 7lb
5ft 7in	9st 6lb	8st 6lb–10st 10lb	12st 12lb
5ft 8in	9st 10lb	8st 10lb–11st 0lb	13st 3lb
5ft 9in	10st 0lb	9st 0lb–11st 4lb	13st 8lb
5ft 10in	10st 4lb	9st 4lb–11st 9lb	14st 0lb
5ft 11in	10st 8lb	9st 8lb–12st 0lb	14st 6lb
6ft 0in	10st 12lb	9st 12lb–12st 5lb	14st 12lb

Women: weight without clothes (kg)
(add 2 kg if you weigh yourself in your clothes)

Height	Average weight	Acceptable weight range	Obese
1.48m	46.5kg	42kg–54kg	65kg
1.50m	47.0kg	43kg–55kg	66kg
1.52m	48.5kg	44kg–57kg	68kg
1.54m	49.5kg	44kg–58kg	70kg
1.56m	50.4kg	45kg–58kg	70kg
1.58m	51.3kg	46kg–59kg	71kg
1.60m	52.6kg	48kg–61kg	73kg
1.62m	54.0kg	49kg–62kg	74kg
1.64m	54.4kg	50kg–64kg	77kg
1.66m	56.8kg	51kg–65kg	78kg
1.68m	58.1kg	52kg–66kg	79kg
1.70m	60.0kg	53kg–67kg	80kg
1.72m	61.3kg	55kg–69kg	83kg
1.74m	62.6kg	56kg–70kg	84kg
1.76m	64.0kg	58kg–72kg	86kg

Tables courtesy of the Scottish Health Education Group

coronary disease have been linked with the number of cups drunk. This association may relate to the other habits that very heavy coffee drinkers tend to have, such as smoking. Nevertheless, it is probably wise to drink no more than 5 cups of coffee a day.

Alcohol

It is widely believed that a little alcohol is good for your coronary arteries; the evidence for this is questionable. However, in moderation it is not harmful to the heart although large quantities certainly are. Useful guidelines are that a woman should not exceed an average of two units a day and a man three (a unit being equivalent to a measure of spirits, a glass of wine or half a pint of beer).

Drugs for reducing cholesterol (see also Chapter 6)

The drugs that have been available for lowering high cholesterol levels in the past have been only mildly effective in this respect, they have quite troublesome side-effects, and they are relatively expensive. Trials with these drugs suggest that they can lead to a substantial reduction in heart attacks and other manifestations of coronary disease, but little or no effect on death rates has been shown. With these facts in mind, it is generally recognized that drug treatment for high lipids should be under-taken only if the level remains high after some months of dietary treat-ment. The exact level at which treatment should be started is still a matter of discussion amongst experts, but certainly if total cholesterol is above 8, few would dispute that drugs are indicated. The development of new drugs that are far more effective in lowering cholesterol and seem relatively free of side-effects may change the principles upon which the prescription of cholesterol-lowering drugs is founded.

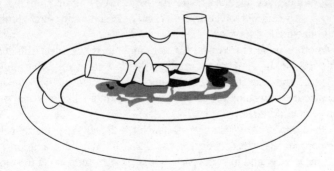

SMOKING

Probably the most important reason for the reduction in coronary deaths in this country and the United States is that so many people have given up cigarettes—it is said there are 11 million ex-smokers in the UK and 35 million in the USA.

The way to a healthy heart

Smoking

DON'T!!! You are harming yourself and those about you. You are providing a bad example to others, especially the young

It's never too late to stop, but the earlier the better. You are protecting yourself against lung cancer as well as coronary disease if you give up

Pipes and cigars may be less dangerous than cigarettes if the smoke is not inhaled, but you still inflict your smoke on others.

Many reasons are given for not stopping smoking. Some people are truly addicted to nicotine; many are not. One excuse is that there is often some increase in weight on giving up—partly because the appetite improves. Some people are sure that smoking makes them relax, but in fact tobacco is a stimulant and makes the heart beat faster. Others think that if they have been smoking for many years, it is too late to stop. This is not the case: whatever age individuals give up smoking, the risk of coronary disease diminishes in the ensuing years but, of course, the earlier one gives up, the greater the benefit. Giving up smoking has a very positive side—food tastes better, breathlessness and cough diminish, and one smells a lot nicer!

Another important reason for not smoking is the effect this has on other people. It is now recognized that 'passive smoking' is harmful, but it is also the case that parents' habits are reflected in their children's behaviour—non-smoking parents are much more likely to have non-smoking children.

Giving up smoking can be very difficult, and help is frequently needed. Supportive relatives can do a great deal, the general practitioner can provide advice, and in some parts of the country there are anti-smoking clinics. Information is available from Action on Smoking and Health

(ASH), 5-11 Mortimer Street, London W1N 7RH (telephone 071 637 9843).

REDUCING HIGH BLOOD PRESSURE

High blood pressure undoubtedly contributes to the development of coronary disease, but trials of blood pressure lowering have been disappointing in their effect on the number of deaths from that disease. This may be because the treatment has not been continued for long enough, or because the blood pressure has not been lowered enough (or too much), or because the drugs used have had adverse effects that have counteracted their benefit. Be that as it may, there are other even more cogent reasons for lowering blood pressure, such as the prevention of stroke and kidney failure.

High blood pressure is first treated without drugs, e.g. by weight reduction, and by reducing alcohol and salt consumption if these seem excessive. If the blood pressure remains high on repeated testing, drugs may be used. Popular drugs include:

- diuretics (which promote the excretion of sodium in the urine);
- calcium antagonists (that relax blood vessels);
- beta-blockers (that counteract the effects of adrenaline and similar hormones that raise the blood pressure);
- ACE inhibitors (that block the angiotensin-converting enzyme (ACE) that leads to the contraction of blood vessels).

All these drugs have side-effects; the doctor has to weigh these up against the potential benefits of treatment in individuals who mostly feel perfectly well. If the blood pressure is only slightly raised, e.g. a systolic pressure

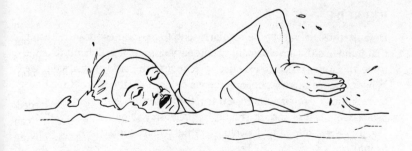

of 150 or a diastolic of 95 (see p. 6), he or she may prefer to delay the administration of drugs to see whether it falls spontaneously. If, however, there are other risk factors for coronary disease or if the blood pressure has already had some adverse effect on the heart or kidneys, more active treatment is necessary.

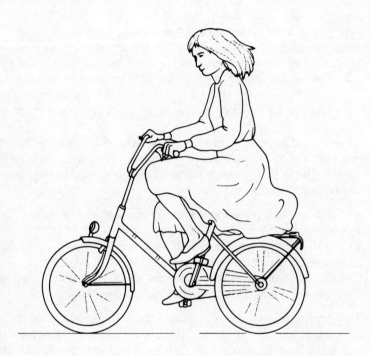

EXERCISE

Because those who exercise regularly tend to have other 'healthy' habits that influence the development of coronary disease, it is difficult to determine the importance of exercise in reducing the risk of heart disease. What evidence there is supports the view that regular (two to three times a week) brisk exercise lasting 20 to 30 minutes on each occasion has a protective effect. Exercise should be preferably dynamic (e.g. walking, jogging, swimming, and cycling) rather than isometric (e.g. weight lifting).

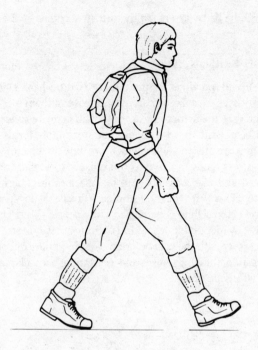

> **The way to a healthy heart**
>
> *Exercise*
>
> Take regular vigorous exercise—it doesn't have to hurt but it should make you slightly breathless
>
> Take it two or three times a week
>
> 20 to 30 minutes per session
>
> Brisk or hill walking, jogging, swimming, cycling, and dancing (but not the slow fox-trot!) are all excellent
>
> Beware squash over 35—unless in good regular training

Squash seems to be a relatively high-risk sport for those over 35 years of age who are not in regular training, particularly if they have a high risk of coronary disease. A sad example of this was Philip Caves, one of the most promising heart surgeons of his day, who died on the squash court at the age of 39; he had a strong family history of coronary disease at an early age.

STRESS AND PERSONALITY

As discussed in the previous chapter, there is little hard evidence to incriminate stress as a cause of coronary disease, although it can undoubtedly aggravate the symptoms of those who actually suffer from it. Common sense suggests that we should minimize those forms of stress that we find distressing and with which we find it difficult to cope. Furthermore, stress tends to make us more likely to smoke and to take unhealthy diets, and may possibly lead to increases in cholesterol and blood pressure. There are many techniques available for controlling stress, and stress counselling is helpful to some people. Most people can help themselves by identifying what kind of things they find stressful and seeking, if necessary with the collaboration of their families or colleagues, ways of combating these. Exercise and relaxation both play a part in reducing the effects of stress.

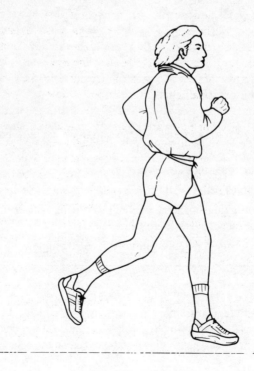

HEALTH SCREENING IN THE PREVENTION
OF CORONARY DISEASE

'Screening' has become very popular in programmes designed to prevent heart disease; it is based on the assumption that if risk factors can be identified, they can be corrected with salutary effects. To be successful, screening must be accurate in identifying the risk factors, reasonably inexpensive, and lead to effective action. It must not, however, cause unnecessary anxiety nor should it inappropriately reassure, as it may well do.

There is widespread agreement about the desirability of detecting some of the risk factors for coronary disease. These include a family history of coronary disease at an early age, smoking habit, overweight, and high blood pressure. It is the province of general practitioners to be aware of such risk factors in their patients, and many now include, in their primary health care team, facilitators whose job it is to ensure that appropriate screening measures of this kind are carried out.

Much more controversial is the measurement of blood cholesterol. Techniques now available allow measurement of blood cholesterol in the doctor's surgery or in the pharmacist's shop from blood obtained by a finger prick. In ideal circumstances, the result of the test done in this way is reasonably accurate but often, either because the apparatus is not well maintained or because of errors in the technique of blood sampling, the results may be grossly inaccurate. Furthermore, there is a variability from time to time in one's blood cholesterol level, so that at least two samples taken at different times are necessary to establish an accurate reading. If the level is indeed found to be raised on repeated sampling, then further investigations need to be undertaken to determine the levels of high density and low density lipoproteins and of triglycerides. The situation is, therefore, more complex and expensive than many appreciate, and the campaign in the United States for everyone to 'know their number' (i.e. their cholesterol level) is a simplistic concept. Even when the number is known, its significance depends very much on the reason for the high level, and on other risk factors. Thus, even with a high cholesterol, the risk of coronary disease is quite low if there are no other risk factors. Simple rules of thumb have been produced, suggesting various strategies depending upon the cholesterol level. Useful as they are, they are very crude guidelines. The figures widely quoted are as follows: above 7.8 the risk of disease is high and drugs are called for if the level does not respond to diet; levels above 6.5 are less serious but still too high and call for stringent dieting; 5.2 is regarded as the target level; cholesterol levels above this and below 6.5 call for a prudent, lipid-lowering diet of the kind outlined above.

If the blood cholesterol is measured, skilled counselling is essential, both because of the need to interpret the result correctly, and because the age and gender of the individual and the other risk factors must be taken into account.

OTHER PREVENTIVE MEASURES

ASPIRIN

There has been interest in the ability of aspirin to prevent heart attacks, particularly since a study on American doctors showed that those taking the drug had a lower incidence of heart attacks. However, only a very small number of attacks was prevented and aspirin may cause a variety of problems including bleeding from the stomach and (very rarely) brain haemorrhages. It is therefore not to be recommended as a routine preventive measure for everyone. Indeed, most doctors would now recommend this drug only for those who are known to have coronary disease. The dose should be small, e.g. one tablet (300 mg) on alternate days or half a tablet daily.

CAUTION WITH THE CONTRACEPTIVE PILL

The relatively low dose oestrogen pills now commonly used impose a negligible risk for the woman who does not have other risk factors. The woman who smokes should give this up rather than stop the pill if she wishes to reduce her risk of coronary disease. However, if there is a strong family history of coronary disease, or if there is high blood pressure, or the cholesterol level is known to be high, it is better to avoid the pill, especially over the age of 35.

HORMONE REPLACEMENT THERAPY (HRT)

The natural female hormones appear to protect the pre-menopausal woman from coronary disease, and it seems reasonable to suppose that the administration of similar hormones to women when they reach the menopause would maintain this protection. Studies with quite high doses of oestrogen appeared to support this concept, but as these seemed to be associated with an increased risk of breast cancer, a lower dose of oestrogen is now often combined with progestogen. Whether this combination protects against coronary disease is not yet known.

Case history—A woman at risk

All her friends were astonished when Sally had a heart attack at the age of 43. She had been the life and soul of the party, and always lavish with the drinks and cigarettes. What they didn't know was that she was still taking an oral contraceptive, and she had an unfortunate family history as both her parents had died in their fifties—her father of a heart attack and her mother of a stroke. When she was investigated by the hospital, it was found that her cholesterol was very high at 9.2 and her blood pressure was slightly raised at 160/96. She was unlucky in having inherited a gene from her father which resulted in the high cholesterol. She should have been advised that, particularly with the bad family history, she should not have smoked and she probably should not have taken the oral contraceptive beyond the age of 35. After the heart attack, she was treated with aspirin and a beta-blocker, and put on a strict, low saturated fat diet. This succeeded in reducing her cholesterol to 8, but her doctor is considering starting her on one of the drugs that lower cholesterol. She has stopped smoking, and made sure that her two brothers and two children (aged 22 and 20) have had their cholesterol levels checked.

5. Tests used in the diagnosis and management of coronary disease

A doctor can learn a great deal about patients with suspected heart disease by simply listening to the description of their complaint and making a physical examination. For example, if a middle-aged man describes a tight pain across the chest that is brought on by exercise and is relieved by rest, one can be almost sure that this is angina, without any special tests. If, however, one wants to be certain of the cause of the symptoms and of the severity of the underlying disease, further tests are necessary. Furthermore, in many cases the features of the case are not typical and tests are necessary to make the diagnosis.

THE ELECTROCARDIOGRAM (ECG)

The ECG is the test most commonly used in the diagnosis of heart disease. It provides a record of the electrical activity of the heart, which is obtained by attaching electrodes (metal plates) to each of the four limbs and to six places on the front and left side of the chest. One feels nothing other than the application of jelly to the chest upon which the electrodes are placed. The test is completely painless and harmless—no electricity goes into the patient from the machine and, in spite of the fears expressed by some patients, there is no danger of an electric shock! The whole procedure can be done in a few minutes in the doctor's surgery or out-patients' department.

The ECG provides a great deal of information about the electrical function of the heart (see Chapter 1), but it does not reveal much about its mechanical (pumping) action. It is possible to see a wave (called the P wave) as the electricity spreads across the atria (Fig. 5.1), but nothing is seen as the current spreads down the very slender tract (the bundle of His) that conducts it through to the ventricles. As the impulse spreads through the ventricles in a rather complicated fashion, it gives rise to what is called the QRS complex. At the end of this time the heart is fully activated; after a short pause, a further flow of current takes place, which returns the heart to the resting state. This final part of the ECG is called

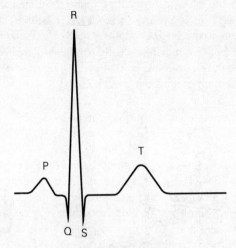

Fig. 5.1. Normal ECG.

the T wave. A particularly important segment is that between the end of the QRS complex and the T wave (called the ST segment) because this is the part of the ECG that is most often affected by coronary disease.

The ECG is very valuable in detecting disturbances of rhythm because it can show irregularities of the heart and, usually, give a clear indication of what is responsible for these.

An ECG is essential in the diagnosis of a heart attack, as it nearly always shows characteristic changes. Early in the attack, however, the ECG may be virtually normal; sometimes the electrocardiographic features are difficult to interpret because of abnormalities that have persisted from a previous heart attack. However, if recordings are taken daily over two or three days, it is nearly always possible to establish whether or not an attack has occurred.

An ECG taken with the patient at rest is often unhelpful in patients with angina, as it may be normal, only revealing changes when exercise is taken. Another important limitation of the ECG is that it may show abnormalities even if the heart is normal.

THE EXERCISE ECG

In many patients with coronary disease there are no symptoms at rest and the ECG is normal. Exercise may bring on both angina and ECG changes—but the ECG abnormalities appear first, and in some cases there is no pain (this is a form of what is called 'silent ischaemia').

Exercise is undertaken either on a treadmill or stationary bicycle. The treadmill consists of a moving belt, the speed and angulation of which can be altered during the test, so that everything from a slow stroll to running uphill can be simulated (Fig. 5.2).

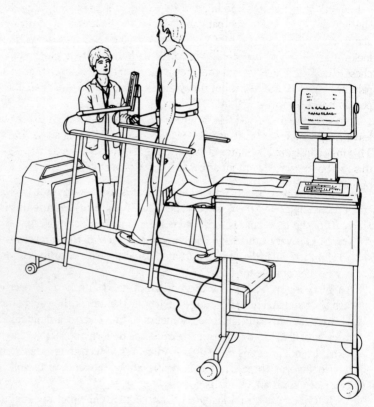

Fig. 5.2. Patient exercising on a treadmill while the ECG is recorded; electrodes are attached to the front of his chest.

Light clothing and shoes (such as trainers) should be worn. Electrodes are attached to the chest and, perhaps, elsewhere on the abdomen and arms. The exercise starts gently, and then every three minutes the amount of work being done is increased, for example, by increasing the speed or the slope of the treadmill. During the test, the ECG is continuously recorded, and a blood pressure reading is obtained every minute. In most cases, the patient is asked to continue the test for as long as possible—this is called a 'maximum symptom-limited' test; the limiting symptom may be angina but normal people are usually stopped by fatigue in the legs or breathlessness. An exercise test usually lasts about 12 to 15 minutes, after which the patient lies down on a couch and recordings are continued for a few minutes.

Frequently, a doctor is standing by at the time of an exercise test; he or she will stop the test if the patient is obviously distressed or if major abnormalities appear on the ECG. What the doctor will be particularly looking for is 'ST depression' (Fig. 5.3). If the patient develops both chest pain and ST depression, this provides convincing evidence that the pain originates in the heart, but if neither occurs it does not exclude the possibility of coronary disease.

A more limited exercise test is now often undertaken before patients leave hospital after a heart attack—perhaps one week after admission. This may consist of 8 minutes of exercise at a speed of 2 miles an hour. If this can be completed without any major symptoms or ECG changes, the outlook is good.

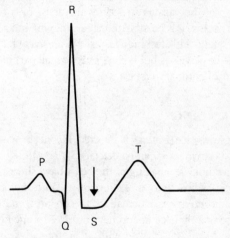

Fig. 5.3. The arrow points to the ST depression of ischaemia—typical of angina (compare this segment with the equivalent part of 5.1).

TAPE RECORDING OF THE ECG

It often happens that patients experience symptoms at home or at work but fail to do so in the doctor's surgery or in hospital. This applies particularly to attacks of palpitation. To overcome this problem, tape recorders have been developed that can record the heart's electrical activity over a 24-hour period. Wires connect electrodes attached to the chest to a small recorder (like a 'Walkman'), which can be worn on a belt around the waist. These recorders are fitted in the hospital ECG department and taken home. They are usually returned the next day. The tape is then removed and analysed (the tape is replayed at high speed, otherwise the ECG technicians would spend a whole day analysing a single tape!). The patient is asked to keep a diary, noting when any symptoms occurred; the tape is then examined with particular care at the corresponding time.

OTHER WAYS OF TESTING THE HEART

ECHOCARDIOGRAPHY

Echocardiography exploits the fact that sound of high frequency (ultrasound) is reflected back when it encounters a boundary between two structures of different densities. The reflected wave can be detected and a picture built up of the various structures traversed by a beam of ultrasound. By this means, it is possible to make a moving image of the heart, painlessly and safely. This technique is used extensively for investigating disorders of the heart valves but it plays only a small part in the diagnosis and assessment of coronary disease.

NUCLEAR IMAGING

If a radioactive substance (isotope) is injected, it concentrates in particular organs and tissues, where it can be detected by a 'gamma camera'. The isotopes used for nuclear imaging of the heart have short half-lives, that is they lose their radioactivity in a short time. With the doses used, the exposure to radioactivity is so small as to constitute no danger. Two types of test are mainly used in coronary disease. In one kind of test the red cells in the blood are labelled with an isotope of technetium. It is possible to assess the way the ventricles are contracting and relaxing by visualizing the changing pattern of the pool of blood cells within them. In the other test, a different isotope (thallium) is used, which is distributed in the muscle of the heart in proportion to the local blood flow. It is therefore possible to detect areas of muscle that receive little or no blood. This test is used particularly in the diagnosis and assessment of angina, as little thallium will reach the area responsible for the angina. The thallium test is usually combined with an exercise test as this tends to accentuate the abnormalities.

CARDIAC CATHETERIZATION

Cardiac catheterization differs from the previous tests in that it is 'invasive', that is it involves the introduction into an artery or vein of a narrow tube (catheter) that is opaque to X-rays. The technique used depends upon exactly what information is sought, but when cardiac catheterization is done on patients with suspected coronary disease, the essential requirement is to visualize the coronary arteries and the left ventricle.

The procedure is carried out in a catheterization laboratory which is equipped with specially designed X-ray apparatus, and various pieces of equipment for monitoring the electrical activity of the heart and recording pressures from within it.

For coronary angiography, the catheter is introduced under a local anaesthetic into an artery either in the front of the elbow or in the groin. The pinprick sensation produced by the needle used for this purpose is the most painful part of the procedure, as the patient is usually unaware of the passage of the catheter into the blood vessels and heart. Once the catheter is introduced, it is advanced up the artery into the aorta where it is kept under visual control by X-ray screening. Experienced operators have little difficulty in directing the tip of the catheter into either of the two coronary arteries or into the left ventricle, particularly as specially shaped catheters are available for each of these sites.

The arteries and left ventricle can be outlined one after the other by selective injection of a radio-opaque fluid, producing what is called an angiogram. This may produce a transient hot flush which can be felt spreading throughout the body.

Because the angiogram is displayed on a large video screen, the picture can be watched by the patient, who is often fascinated by it. It is possible to visualize the location of any narrowings in the coronary arteries (Fig. 5.4), and also to see whether there are parts of the left ventricle which are not contracting as well as they should.

When the catheter is withdrawn, it is necessary to put in some stitches if it was inserted in the arm, or to compress the artery in the groin for about 10 minutes if this has been used. The affected limb should be rested for some hours after the investigation.

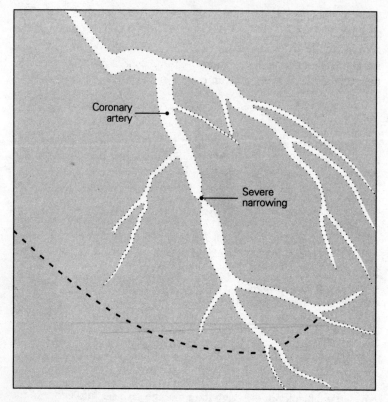

Fig. 5.4. The demonstration of coronary artery narrowing by coronary angiography.

Cardiac catheterization does entail some discomfort, and even some risk, so it is undertaken only if it is felt that the information it provides is necessary for the management of the patient. It is absolutely essential in deciding upon the need for angioplasty (see p. 62) or surgery as it is the only technique that allows a precise delineation of the narrowings of the coronary arteries.

The commonest complications are bruising in the groin or a weak pulse in the arm. These may cause some discomfort for a few days, and necessitate keeping the affected limb at rest during that period. Serious complications can occur, of which the most important is that of a heart attack which could be fatal. The risk of this is about one in a thousand, but such problems are largely confined to those who have the most advanced forms of the disease and are most in need of urgent treatment.

The risk to someone who has been in relatively good health is very much smaller.

In most cases, a patient is admitted to hospital for the procedure, but increasingly cardiac catheterizations are being done on a 'day case' basis, thereby reducing the need for an overnight stay.

6. Treatment

The management of coronary disease includes advice about necessary changes in diet, smoking, and the way of life, but sooner or later nearly all patients need drugs, and many will benefit from such interventions as angioplasty and surgery. This chapter describes for a patient the various drugs available, the ways in which they are used, and their potential adverse effects, as well as the diagnosis and treatment of a cardiac arrest. It also recounts what is involved when undergoing angioplasty or surgery.

DRUGS

The drugs used specifically for the management of coronary disease fall into three main groups:

- anti-anginal drugs—nitrates, beta-blockers, calcium antagonists (Table 6.1);
- drugs for preventing or treating thrombosis—aspirin and other 'anti-platelet' drugs, anticoagulants, thrombolytic drugs;
- lipid-lowering drugs—fibrates, nicotinic acid, resins, enzyme inhibitors.

In addition to these categories of drug that are used for the direct treatment of coronary disease, there are many that are used to treat conditions which complicate coronary disease or are associated with it, such as heart failure, rhythm disturbances, and high blood pressure. It is not proposed to discuss all these here because there are so many of them. The trade names of many cardiac drugs are listed at the end of this chapter.

ANTI-ANGINAL DRUGS

Nitrates

Nitrates have been used for the treatment of angina for more than a hundred years, and are still often prescribed for this condition. More

Table 6.1. Anti-anginal drugs

	Uses	Side-effects
Nitrates	Angina Heart failure	Headache, dizziness, faintness, fainting
Beta-blockers	Angina Preventing heart attacks High blood pressure Rhythm disorders	Fatigue, tiredness, lethargy, aggravation of heart failure and asthma, cold extremities, and other less common problems
Calcium antagonists	Angina High blood pressure	Flushing, headaches, swollen ankles, gastric upsets, constipation, dizziness, fainting

For trade names, see the end of this chapter.

recently, they have been used in the treatment of heart failure. Their main action is to relax the muscles in the walls of veins and arteries (including the coronary arteries); their most important action is probably the relaxation of veins, as this reduces the amount of blood returning to the heart and thereby the work that it has to do. This action is especially important in heart failure, but their ability to relax the coronary arteries is of value in coronary artery spasm.

A particular problem with nitrates is the development of tolerance—that is the loss of effect with continued use. This occurs if they are continuously present in the blood; it is now usual to ensure that there is some period during the 24 hours which is 'nitrate-free'.

Numerous preparations are available which are given in a variety of different contexts.

Glyceryl trinitrate (also called GTN, trinitrin, and nitroglycerin)
Glyceryl trinitrate is issued to almost all anginal patients as it relieves the discomfort very quickly and is particularly effective in preventing an expected attack. The tablet should be put under the tongue and allowed to dissolve there—it becomes inactive if swallowed. It can cause a fierce, throbbing headache, particularly when first tried, but this tends to

diminish or disappear with continued use. It can also produce flushing, dizziness, or even fainting; when first used, it is advisable to sit or lie down to see the reaction. The tablets tend to deteriorate with use and should be disposed of if unused after six to eight weeks. The active ingredient can be absorbed by cotton wool and they are best kept in a glass container with a foil-lined cap, without any cotton wool wadding.

Another way of administering glyceryl trinitrate is by *aerosol spray*. Two metered doses should be sprayed on or under the tongue. The canister should not be shaken and caution is necessary (particularly with smokers) as the spray is inflammable.

Buccal nitrates are tablets that gradually release the drug over four to six hours if positioned between the upper lip and gum.

Several preparations of nitrates are active when *swallowed*, such as isosorbide mononitrate and dinitrate. A popular form of nitrate is the *self-adhesive patch*, usually placed on the chest wall 'over the heart'. If given in sufficient dosage, enough of the drug is absorbed through the skin to relieve or prevent angina. The attempt to provide '24-hour cover' with these patches has, however, proved unsuccessful because of the development of tolerance, but they do have a powerful placebo effect if placed in the right spot!

Nitrates can also be given by *intravenous infusion* in emergencies such as unstable angina, myocardial infarction, and heart failure.

Side-effects   The side-effects of flushing, headache, and faintness are greatest with sublingual glyceryl trinitrate but occur to a greater or lesser extent with all the nitrates.

Beta-blockers

Their full name is beta-adrenergic receptor-blocking agents (or beta-adrenoceptor-blocking agents). These drugs block the effects of hormones such as adrenaline which increase the heart rate and the vigour with which it contracts. Exercise and emotion often cause the heart to beat faster and more forcefully than it really needs; beta-blocking drugs damp down these effects and reduce the heart's need for oxygen. Because of these actions, beta-blockers have been used by perfectly healthy people whose professional performance may be affected by anxiety, such as musicians and snooker players. Beta-blockers are very effective in combating angina when it is caused by exertion or emotion. They work too slowly to be effective in an attack of angina, but they are very valuable in preventing attacks coming on. They reduce the risk of a further heart attack or death in those who have already had one heart attack. Another important action of beta-blockers is to lower blood pressure and they are frequently used in the treatment of hypertension.

Side-effects In some people, these drugs can reduce the heart rate or blood pressure too much, and they should not be given to patients who already have a slow heart rate or low blood pressure. They can also adversely affect the pumping action of the heart and aggravate heart failure. Other undesirable effects are that they may cause constriction of the air passages (bronchi) and may mask the symptoms of low blood sugar. They should be used with great caution in asthmatics and in diabetics on insulin treatment; some beta-blockers are classified as 'selective' because they act almost exclusively on the heart, but they too must be used with great care in patients at risk of their various adverse effects. All the more serious adverse effects of beta-blockers are uncommon when used in patients without the problems just mentioned. On the other hand, minor ones, such as lethargy, tiredness, fatigue, and cold extremities, are frequent; rarely there may be nausea, diarrhoea, impotence or other sexual disorders, or pins and needles in the fingers.

Calcium antagonists

A regular influx of calcium into the muscle cells of the heart and blood vessels is essential for their contraction. The calcium antagonists (or calcium blockers) limit the amount of calcium that goes into the muscle cells. They relax the arteries (including the coronary arteries), and in so doing increase the blood supply to the heart and reduce the work it has to do to pump blood through the circulation. These drugs are used in the treatment of angina and high blood pressure and are most often given regularly once to three times a day by mouth, but for a quick effect during an attack of angina, a nifedipine capsule may be bitten through and its contents retained in the mouth. Some of the calcium antagonists (e.g. verapamil and diltiazem) affect the electrical activity of the heart, tending to slow its rate and being useful in the treatment of some types of rhythm disturbance. Others (such as nifedipine and nicardipine) have no such effect, and indeed make the heart beat faster. Perhaps because of this, very occasionally angina may be provoked by these two preparations. Calcium antagonists have a special role when coronary spasm or increased tension in the muscular walls of the coronary arteries are an important factor in angina, and when angina and high blood pressure coexist. They are, however, often used effectively in the treatment of angina due to exercise. All the calcium antagonists have the capacity of causing a deterioration in the pumping action of the heart, especially when this is already poor. Although not often a problem, doctors usually avoid giving these drugs to patients with heart failure.

Side-effects Calcium antagonists are usually well tolerated and dangerous side-effects are rare. Verapamil can cause troublesome constipation, and they all may cause a variety of gastro-intestinal disturbances. Because they relax blood vessels, patients quite often experience flushing and headache; other side-effects include dizziness and faintness and swelling of the ankles. Unlike the beta-blockers, they do not have adverse effects in asthmatics and diabetics. Because beta-blockers slow the heart, they are seldom given together with verapamil and diltiazem, but their combination with nifedipine or nicardipine is a particularly advantageous one.

The choice and combination of anti-anginal drugs

All three kinds of anti-anginal drug are effective, but individuals differ, often unpredictably, in their responsiveness to them and in the side-effects they experience. The first drug that a doctor chooses to treat angina depends both upon the characteristics of the individual patient and upon the doctor's own preferences. Thus, for example, beta-blockers are generally avoided in asthmatics and in diabetics who require insulin, but they are the preferred drugs in patients who have had a heart attack because they reduce the risk of further attacks. Curiously, there are major differences in the use of the various drugs in different countries, beta-blockers being particularly popular in the UK and Scandinavia, while the calcium antagonists are more in vogue in the United States and Italy. The combination of two or three drugs, each from a different type, may achieve greater success in relieving the symptoms while reducing the side-effects.

DRUGS USED TO PREVENT OR TREAT CLOTTING OF THE BLOOD
Aspirin
Aspirin has been used as a pain-relieving drug for more than a hundred years, but only recently has it been realized that it is very effective in preventing the clotting of blood. It does this by preventing the clumping together of the platelet cells in the blood, which is usually the first stage

of the clotting process (see p. 00). It is still uncertain what the best dose of aspirin is as, theoretically, large doses might actually increase the danger of clotting. The most common dosage now used is one-half to one 300–325 mg tablet daily, but the 75 mg tablet is becoming popular.

Aspirin is now of proven value in and after acute heart attacks, in unstable angina, and in patients with coronary artery bypass vein grafts (see below). Less sure is its place in patients with chronic angina and in apparently healthy middle-aged men who are at risk of heart attack. One has to weigh up the risks of the drug, albeit small, against the benefits.

Side-effects Aspirin can cause or aggravate bleeding from the gut, cause dyspepsia, nausea, vomiting, and constipation and, very rarely, a brain haemorrhage. The stomach problems can in some people be overcome by using buffered or enteric-coated (e.g. Nu-Seals) aspirin. Very occasionally, aspirin can precipitate asthma.

Other 'anti-platelet' drugs

Other drugs with similar actions may be used instead of aspirin, or in addition to it. These include dipyridamole (Persantin) and sulphin-pyrazone (Anturan). Dipyridamole is taken by mouth three or four times a day. It is usually well tolerated, but should be taken at least one hour before meals to avoid the dyspepsia that may occur. Other occasional side-effects include dizziness, flushing, faintness, mild diarrhoea, and rash, and, very seldom, an aggravation of angina. Sulphinpyrazone is taken by mouth once to three times a day. It may cause disturbances of the kidneys and blood, which necessitate periodic blood tests; sometimes it precipitates gout in those susceptible to it. It may also cause dyspepsia and, very occasionally, bleeding from the gut. Both these drugs have to be used with great care if anticoagulants are being given.

Anticoagulants

Anticoagulant drugs prevent the formation of clots, not by their action on platelets, but by preventing the precipitation of fibrin, the protein component of clots.

Heparin

This drug is usually given intravenously, but sometimes subcutaneously. It is used when there is an urgent need to prevent clotting or to prevent the spreading of a clot already present. It is therefore often given for

unstable angina or after a heart attack, particularly if the patient is kept
in bed, in order to prevent clots in the legs which are common in the
immobile, and which may, in turn, lead to clots in the lungs. It is seldom
used for more than seven days before changing to oral anticoagulants.

Oral anticoagulants

Warfarin is the most commonly used oral anticoagulant and may be
given for months or years if there is a continuing risk of thrombosis. It is
especially valuable when there has been clotting in the veins in the legs,
or in the lungs or within the heart itself. There is a major risk of bleeding
when warfarin is given, so it is necessary for it to be closely controlled by
periodic blood tests, and patients need to be warned to take the precise
dose prescribed and to beware of the various drugs that may reduce or
increase its activity. Amongst numerous drugs which interact with
warfarin are aspirin, cimetidine (Tagamet) and agents used in the treatment of arthritis, gout, epilepsy, high blood cholesterol, and disorders of
heart rhythm. If given to pregnant women, it may damage the fetus.

Its activity is monitored by regular blood tests that measure what is
called the 'International Normalized Ratio' (INR), which compares the
time taken for the patient's blood to clot with a standard; this may be
referred to as the 'prothrombin time' or some similar expression. The
dosage of warfarin is adjusted on the basis of this test, which may be done
almost every day initially, but perhaps every four to six weeks eventually.

Thrombolytic drugs

Drugs that dissolve (lyse) the fibrin in clots are known as thrombolytic or
fibrinolytic drugs or, in popular usage 'clot-busters'. Although they may
have a place in the management of a number of conditions due to clots, it
is in the treatment of heart attacks due to coronary thrombosis (myocardial infarction) that they have an outstandingly important role. Large
trials of these drugs in hospitals have shown that they can reduce the
likelihood of death from a heart attack by 25 to 50 per cent. The most
commonly used agent is streptokinase; newer drugs include alteplase
(Actilyse) and anistreplase (Eminase). Alteplase—also known as rt-PA
(recombinant tissue plasminogen activator)—has excited particular
interest because it is a substance that occurs naturally in the tissues of
the human body but can be manufactured by 'genetic engineering'.
It has the advantage of not causing allergic reactions, as the other
thrombolytic drugs may do, but it is expensive and has not been shown
to be more effective and safer than its rivals. However, because it does

not cause allergic reactions it can be used for second attacks whereas streptokinase and anistreplase can do so and should not be repeated within a year. Alteplase is given by an intravenous infusion (drip) over three hours, whereas streptokinase is infused over one hour, and anistreplase injected into a vein within five minutes. All these agents may cause excessive bleeding and are avoided in patients known to be at risk of this—for example, those with stomach ulcers or recent stroke, trauma or surgery. To be most effective, these drugs need to be given as soon as possible after the beginning of a heart attack.

DRUGS FOR HIGH BLOOD FATS ('LIPID-LOWERING DRUGS')

High levels of fats or lipids (e.g. cholesterol) in the blood should always be treated by diet first (see Chapter 4) but when this alone fails, drugs with a lipid-lowering action may be given (Table 6.2).

Cholestyramine (Questran) and colestipol (Colestid) are *resin* drugs which are not absorbed from the gut but act there on the bile in such a way that more cholesterol is broken down to bile in the liver and

Table 6.2. Drugs for lowering cholesterol

Class of drug	Names	Side-effects
Resins	Cholestyramine (Questran) Colestipol (Colestid)	Granules in sachets unpleasant to take; gastric upsets, constipation
Fibrates	Bezafibrate (Bezalip-Mono) Clofibrate (Atromid-S) Fenofibrate (Lipantil) Gemfibrozil (Lopid)	Gastric upsets, muscle cramps
Nicotinic acid derivatives	Acipimox (Olbetam) Nicofuranose (Bradilan)	Flushing, dizziness, stomach upset, liver damage
Statins: enzyme inhibitors	Simvastatin (Zocor) Pravastatin (Lipostat)	Stomach upsets, muscle pains, fatigue, rash, headache

NB. New drugs are constantly coming on to the market.
Only the commoner side-effects are listed here—always inform your doctor of any new symptoms that might be due to a drug.

therefore removed. These drugs come in the form of granules in sachets. They should not be taken dry, but mixed with water or other fluids (such as orange juice or soups). Many patients find them unpleasant to take, and they may cause a variety of gastro-intestinal symptoms, especially constipation (which is usually transient).

Nicotinic acid acts on the liver to prevent the formation of fats. It frequently causes unpleasant symptoms, including flushing, dizziness, and palpitation. The flushing can be diminished by taking aspirin. Rarely, it can result in liver damage.

Clofibrate (Atromid-S), bezafibrate (Bezalip), and gemfibrozil (Lopid) are known as *fibrates* and work primarily by breaking down the tri-glycerides, with relatively slight effects on cholesterol. Large trials of clofibrate and gemfibrozil have shown that they reduce the risk of heart attacks in patients with high fat levels, but may cause a number of problems including gall-stones and other gastro-intestinal disorders.

A new group of drugs—sometimes called the '*statins*' (such as simvastatin [Zocor])—block the production of cholesterol by the liver and have profound effects on the level of cholesterol in the blood. Experience with them is relatively short as yet, but they can lead to a 25 to 40 per cent reduction in cholesterol, with comparatively few side-effects. If trials now in progress confirm their safety and efficacy, they are likely to become the drugs of choice in treating high blood fat levels.

CARDIAC ARREST AND CARDIOPULMONARY RESUSCITATION

There are probably some 60 000 sudden deaths a year in the UK as a consequence of coronary disease; possibly 20 000 of these could be prevented if everyone knew how to do cardiopulmonary resuscitation (CPR) and if all emergency ambulances had well-trained personnel and a defibrillator. A description of CPR follows, but this is no substitute for a formal training programme, which every adolescent and adult should undergo, more especially those with relatives or colleagues with heart disease.

A cardiac arrest is usually the result of a chaotic heart rhythm called *ventricular fibrillation*. In this disorder, the electrical activity of the heart becomes completely disorganized, and the heart stops pumping blood. Less often, the electrical activity of the heart stops altogether—'asystole'. In either case, consciousness is lost quickly and, if the circulation is not restored in some way in three to four minutes, irreparable brain damage will occur.

A cardiac arrest can be diagnosed if an unconscious person has no pulse. It is best to check first that the patient is truly unconscious by giving him or her a shake, and shouting 'are you all right?' If there is no response, one should shout for help and start CPR. The essential features of this are summarized by 'ABC', A being for airway, B for breathing and C for circulation.

Airway. If the individual is to survive, he or she must receive air into the lungs and blood must be circulating, but the first manoeuvre is to ensure that the airway to the lungs is open. This is achieved by tilting the chin forward and preventing the tongue falling back in the throat. To do this, two fingers are used to lift the chin.

Breathing. Sometimes with a cardiac arrest, breathing continues for a short while, but usually it stops within a few seconds. If the subject has stopped breathing, the next step is to give two breaths by the mouth-to-mouth technique. This is done by placing one's mouth over the opened mouth of the patient, while pinching their nose and keeping the chin tilted upwards.

Circulation. If after these two breaths there is still no response, the pulse should be checked. The easiest pulse to feel is the carotid in the neck; two fingers should be put in the groove between the side of the Adam's apple and the large muscle that runs from the angle of the jaw to the front of the collar bone. The fingers should be applied firmly, and if no pulse can be felt, one should assume there is a cardiac arrest and start chest compression. This is done by kneeling by the side of the patient, and finding the lower end of the breastbone (sternum). The heel of one hand is then placed a short distance above this. The heel of the other hand is positioned on top of the first, the shoulders being over the chest and the arms in a vertical position with the elbows straight (Fig. 6.1). The chest is compressed one to two inches firmly, and then released promptly, 80 times a minute.

Both respiration and circulation have to be maintained, a difficult but not impossible task if one is alone. In this circumstance, 15 compressions should be alternated with two breaths. If two people are available, one breath should be given to each five compressions.

It is possible to keep patients alive for a considerable period with well-performed CPR, but if ventricular fibrillation is the cause of the cardiac arrest, a defibrillator will be required. Many ambulances now have these, as do a number of general practitioners. Transferring the patient to hospital as quickly as possible is a priority.

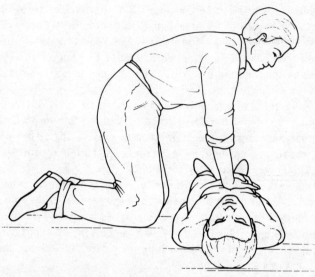

Fig. 6.1. Cardiopulmonary resuscitation, showing the technique of chest compression.

The ABC OF CPR

Airway: lift the chin forward to keep the tongue from falling back
Breathing: mouth-to-mouth resuscitation ('the kiss of life')
Circulation: check the pulse in the neck (carotid pulse)
   If absent, assume there is cardiac arrest and start chest compression

---

ANGIOPLASTY

The technique of percutaneous transluminal coronary angioplasty (PTCA)—often called balloon angioplasty—was introduced in 1977 and is now in widespread use. It has an established place as an alternative to surgery, and has the advantages of avoiding the problems of a major operation, being less expensive, usually requiring only two or three days in hospital, and allowing a quicker return to normal life. Essentially, the procedure is one of introducing into an artery through the skin (i.e. percutaneously) a specially designed catheter which is advanced through the aorta to the lumen of the narrowed coronary artery. Close to the tip of the catheter is an uninflated sausage-shaped balloon which is then inflated at the site of the narrowing so as to stretch the artery and leave it with a wider bore (Fig. 6.2).

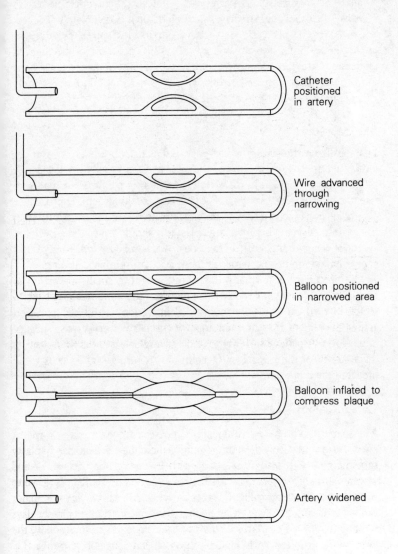

Catheter
positioned
in artery

Wire advanced
through
narrowing

Balloon positioned
in narrowed area

Balloon inflated to
compress plaque

Artery widened

Fig. 6.2. The technique of angioplasty.

Preparation

Before undertaking this procedure, a coronary angiogram (see p. 49) must be done to locate the narrowing and to determine whether it is suitable for angioplasty. An artery may not be suitable for a variety of reasons, such as if the narrowing is too long or it is completely blocked. Some 20 to 30 per cent of coronary narrowings appear suitable, on angiographic films, for angioplasty; about 90 per cent of attempts at angioplasty are successful in widening the vessel. Angioplasty has been used chiefly when only one coronary artery is narrowed, but increasingly it is being used when two or three arteries are involved.

The procedure

Like cardiac catheterization (see p. 49), it is usually undertaken under local anaesthesia to the groin; the patient is normally well sedated. Inflation of the balloon in the artery is frequently painless but may give rise to a brief episode of angina. Patients can usually watch the procedure on a television screen if they wish. Sue Townsend (of *Adrian Mole* fame) has written of seeing her own angioplasty 'It should have won a BAFTA award, it was riveting stuff' in her book *Mr Bevan's dream*. Many other people have found the experience more fascinating than daunting.

The procedure is normally uneventful, but in a small proportion of cases, instead of opening the artery it may lead to a complete obstruction, which in turn can lead to a myocardial infarction. If this complication arises, the patient may need emergency coronary artery bypass surgery (see below). A patient agreeing to undergo angioplasty must therefore be made aware of the possibility of going on to surgery, and needs to be prepared for this eventuality.

Complications

Most patients who have an angioplasty have the procedure days or weeks after the original coronary angiogram, when the cardiologist has had time to review the films, perhaps with a cardiac surgeon, to decide whether angioplasty or surgery is the better option. Usually, it is planned to take place when a cardiac surgeon is available in case of any complications. Increasingly, however, angioplasty is carried out immediately after the angiogram, particularly if this has been done as an emergency, for example in patients with unstable angina that has not responded to medical treatment.

Results

Angioplasty will relieve angina in most cases, but there is a risk in about
a quarter of cases that the artery may narrow again in the succeeding six
months; a further angioplasty is then usually successful, as in the case of
Simon D. He had been quite well until, at the age of 52, he developed
chest pain on a walking holiday in Scotland. Over the next three weeks,
the pain came on with less and less exertion until it started coming on at
rest. He was taken into hospital in Edinburgh. When the pain had settled
down, a coronary angiogram was done, which showed that one of his
coronary arteries was severely narrowed. An angioplasty was very
successful and he had no further pain until four months later, when the
angina came back. A further angioplasty was done, and he has remained
well for the last three years.

New techniques of angioplasty are being developed, such as combining
it with laser treatment, but these must still be regarded as experimental.

CORONARY ARTERY BYPASS SURGERY

Coronary artery bypass graft operations (also known as CABG or,
unfortunately, 'cabbage'!) were first introduced in 1968 and have
proved enormously successful. Such operations are now the commonest
form of major surgery of any kind, about 200 000 being performed each
year in the United States and perhaps some 15 000 in the UK. The
purpose of the operation is to bypass narrowings in the coronary arteries
by inserting a new blood vessel between the aorta and the affected
coronary artery beyond the narrowing. Most often, this is done by taking
a piece of vein from one or other leg, and sewing one end to the aorta and
the other to the coronary artery (Fig. 6.3). It is possible to deal with
several arteries: frequently, three vessels are treated in this way, but
sometimes up to six grafts are inserted. Alternatively, an internal
mammary (thoracic) artery is used. In this case, as the artery is already
attached to the aorta, this attachment is left in place, but the far end is
cut and attached to the relevant coronary artery.

The decision on which and how many arteries are to be operated upon
is determined by the coronary angiogram. To be successful, there has to
be an open artery of adequate size beyond the last narrowing; sometimes
an artery may be completely blocked and impossible to graft.

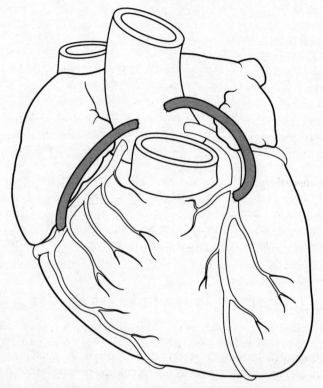

Fig. 6.3. Coronary artery bypass surgery: grafts (stippled) join the aorta to the anterior descending artery and the right coronary artery.

Every operation carries a risk, but coronary bypass surgery is one of the safest of the major operations. The risk of death from the operation is about 1 per cent in a 'good risk' patient, that is, one who has not had a severe heart attack and has no other important medical problem. Complications of the operation include phlebitis (inflammation of the veins related to the operation on the leg), wound infection, and, very rarely, a stroke.

Preparation

The surgeon needs to have a good view of the heart and to be able to reach almost all parts of it. To do this, the breastbone has to be split from top to bottom—this is called 'midline sternotomy'. Sterility is extremely important and the chest wall has to be cleaned very meticulously before the operation; to help this it is necessary to shave the chest in men. Because the legs may be used to take grafts, and the groin region for the insertion of tubes, the legs and groin regions are also shaved (sometimes by the patient him- or herself).

The patient has to refrain from food or drink for a number of hours before the operation. Sedation ('pre-med') as a tablet or injection may be given some time before going to the anaesthetic room, to which the patient is taken on a trolley. By this time, the patient feels very sleepy but is usually aware of a needle being put into the hand or arm and may be given oxygen through a mask gently put on the face by the anaesthetist.

The operation
The patient may be in the operating theatre for one to three hours or more, depending mainly upon the number of grafts that are being used. During the operation, the patient is connected to a heart–lung machine (cardiopulmonary bypass). Blood flows out of the body through tubes put into the large veins and passes through an oxygenator before being returned into the aorta.

After the operation
After the operation, the patient is taken to the intensive care unit (ICU). Anyone who has watched medical programmes on television has some idea of what such a unit is like, but real life is rather different from the frenetic activity as depicted by the media (Fig. 6.4). It is true that patients are usually lying flat and unconscious, and are attached by a variety of tubes and wires to machines (monitors) which display the electrocardiogram (which may 'beep' from time to time) and other signals of bodily function, but the atmosphere is one of calm efficiency. Dramas are rare, but patients are very closely observed in the first few hours after the operation for any untoward features, which are promptly corrected.

A catheter has to be placed in the bladder to monitor the amount of urine being produced, and tubes in the arteries and veins permit close observation of the blood pressure and the delivery of drugs. Tubes go through the chest wall to drain away any fluid that might develop in the chest, but the tube that is most resented is that going through the mouth into the larynx to ensure that ventilation of the lungs is guaranteed; it is usually linked to an artificial ventilator for several hours or even days after the operation. This tube is taken out as soon as the doctors are sure that the patient's own breathing is adequate. It would be alarming to find so many tubes coming out of one's body if no warning had been given,

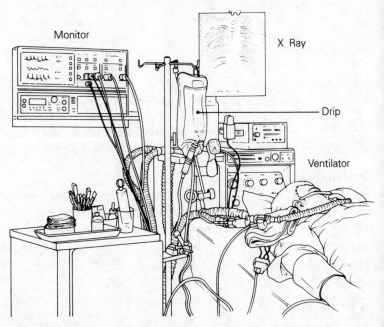

Fig. 6.4. A patient in an intensive care unit. The patient is being artificially ventilated, with tubes going from his windpipe to a ventilator; his heart rhythm and blood pressure are being monitored.

but patients are told before the operation that these are all part of the routine.

Inevitably there is some discomfort in the wounds immediately after the operation, but this is usually controlled very effectively by drugs. After the coronary bypass operation it may be possible to leave the ICU on the day of the operation or the next day, but occasionally a longer stay is necessary.

Within a day or two of the operation, the patient is often feeling surprisingly well, and can start sitting out of bed. The pain in the region of the scars in the chest and leg persists for some time, but there may also be numbness in these regions. Coughing can be very unpleasant and sneezing sheer hell; if someone can hold the chest back and front during coughing this helps a lot. If there is no one to help, coughing is easier if one hugs a pillow or, better, a large teddy bear! Physiotherapists play an important role in helping patients to breathe and cough after the operation, and also in getting them back on their feet.

Getting up

Mobilization starts with short walks around the bed or around the ward on the second or third day after surgery; before going home most patients have gone up and down one or two flights of stairs. It is not a good idea to spend much time sitting in an armchair with one's legs hanging down; this encourages swelling of the legs, particularly if a vein has been removed from one. Soon after the operation, standing still may bring on faint feelings, particularly when showering. It is a good idea to ensure that there is a stool or chair at hand. Because of the problem of swelling of the legs, special elastic stockings are used; these may be needed for several weeks and the patient needs to be instructed in how best to use them. Patients may also experience discomfort in the shoulder region as well as the chest; this is due to manipulation of the chest wall at the time of surgery.

Eating, drinking, and the bowels

It is usual for the appetite to disappear after a major operation, and the first meals should be very light. On the other hand, it is common to be thirsty, but it is better to take frequent small drinks rather than large ones. Intravenous drips are used to prevent dehydration but can usually be taken down when adequate fluids are being taken by mouth. Constipation is almost the rule after surgery and can be distressing. It can usually be overcome by a mild laxative.

Depression and other mental problems

Depression is a major bugbear after surgery. Often, the first two or three days are a time of euphoria, when the patient rejoices in the fact that he or she has come through the experience so well. Then, often in hospital but sometimes not until after return home, gloom descends for no obvious reason. This clears up in a few days, but it is best for patients and their relatives to be prepared for it and to recognize that it will be a transient affair.

Other mental problems may also occur, particularly a temporary impairment of memory, and occasionally there is a period of confusion or hallucination, or a visual disturbance. Less often, there are more serious disturbances of brain function, including very rarely, a stroke. With modern techniques these complications are becoming less common.

Going home

For most patients, this is a giant step forward, but one that they and their relatives may be apprehensive about. This is partly because the patient has been in a protected environment and has been able to call upon expert doctors or nurses at any time if any problem should arise. In fact, if things are taken progressively, return to a normal life is usually un-interrupted. However, the patient must expect to experience discomfort in the chest and leg (if the latter has been operated upon). There is often a slight discharge from the wound, which is quite normal, but needs attention if there is a great deal of it. Swelling of the operated leg can be troublesome, and the numbness and pain may be more annoying than the chest wound itself. It is very important to put the support stocking on before getting out of bed in the morning when the leg is at its slimmest.

Exercise

Exercise is the key to recovery after coronary bypass surgery, but it must be undertaken sensibly. For the first two or three days, it should be no more than was prescribed in hospital, but thereafter it can be increased day by day until quite long walks are being taken, provided the weather is good enough. Some people feel that they should get back to gardening and housework as soon as possible, but the chest wound means that such things as lifting or polishing are very uncomfortable. These kinds of activity are often started with enthusiasm and then rapidly abandoned. Another problem is tiredness. This is a normal reaction to a major operation, but it can be distressing and is a factor in the depression that so often occurs.

Pain

Coronary bypass surgery usually abolishes angina, but it does not always do so completely. It can then be difficult for the patient to know whether any chest pain is due to the wound or comes from the heart. If it really is angina, it is likely to come on only with exercise and be quickly relieved by rest or glyceryl trinitrate. Wound pain is also aggravated by exercise, but particularly by arm movements or lifting, and is brought on by pressure on the chest or coughing. Another type of pain which may be confusing is that from the gullet. People who are liable to get heartburn from the regurgitation of acid into their gullet sometimes find it is worse after lying in bed for a long time, but this pain is usually distinguished by the fact that it is made worse by lying flat, especially after a large meal.

Sexual activity

There is often a great deal of anxiety about returning to sexual activity after surgery, particularly if this has caused angina in the past. The main impediment to intercourse after surgery is, in fact, the chest wound, and it is important to try and find a position where this does not cause discomfort. Generally speaking, it is some three to four weeks after the operation before the patient feels ready to resume sexual activity. Even then there may be some difficulty—there may be a period of impotence in males, but this usually resolves in the succeeding weeks.

Driving

With a successful bypass operation, there is no real bar to driving but it is better not to start too soon. The driving position may be quite uncomfortable and it may be impossible or extremely painful to undertake the sudden manoeuvres that may be necessary to avoid an accident.

Diet, smoking, and drinking

Diet is important after bypass surgery—it has been found that grafts are more likely to close off if the blood cholesterol level is high. Likewise, smoking must be strictly avoided for ever. Alcohol in moderation is not harmful to the heart; many patients find after returning home that a glass of wine or beer is particularly enjoyable.

Medication

Although one of the benefits of surgery is the fact that many medicines that were previously necessary are no longer required, some medication is nearly always prescribed. This is most often aspirin, but may include anticoagulants, or drugs for treating blood pressure or high cholesterol. Occasionally, it is necessary to have anti-anginal drugs, but usually much less than before the operation.

NAMES OF DRUGS USED IN TREATING CORONARY DISEASE

ANTI-ANGINAL DRUGS

Nitrates

Cardiacap, Cedocard retard, Coro-Nitro, Deponit, Elantan, Glyceryl trinitrate, Imdur, Ismo, Isoket retard, Isordil, Isotrate, MCR 50, Monit, Mono-Cedocard, Mycardol, Nitrocine, Nitrocontin Continus, Nitrolingual, Percutol, Soni-slo, Sorbichew, Sorbid SA, Sorbitrate, Suscard Buccal, Sustac, Transiderm-Nitro, Vascardin

Beta-blockers
Atenolol, Bedranol, Berkolol, Beta-Cardone, Betaloc, Betim, Blocadren, Cartrol, Corgard, Emcor, Inderal LA, Labetalol, Lopresor, Metoprolol, Monocor, Oxprenolol, Propranolol, Sectral, Slow-Pren, Slow-Trasicor, Sotacor, Tenormin, Trandate, Trasicor, Visken

Calcium antagonists
Adalat, Adizem Continus, Angiozem, Britiazim, Calcilat, Cardene, Coracten, Cordilox, Istin, Nifedipine, Securon, Tildiem, Univer, Verapamil

Combined beta-blocker and calcium antagonist
Beta-Adalat, Tenif

DRUGS THAT AFFECT BLOOD CLOTTING

Anticoagulants
Calciparine, Dindevan, Marevan, Minihep, Monoparin, Multiparin, Sinthrome, Uniparin

Aspirin
Angettes, Nu-seals, Platet 300

Other anti-platelet drugs
Persantin, Anturan

Fibrinolytic (clot-busting) drugs
Actilyse, Eminase, Kabikinase, Streptase, Streptokinase

LIPID-LOWERING DRUGS

Fibrates
Atromid-S, Bezalip, Lipantil, Lopid

Bile acid sequestrants
Colestid, Questran

'Statin' (HMG CoA reductase inhibitor)
Lipostat, Zocor

Other lipid lowering drugs
Bradilan, Lurselle, Maxepa, Olbetam

DIURETICS

Diuretics are used widely in the treatment of heart failure and of high blood pressure. They work by increasing the amount of sodium in the urine, but some also increase the amount of potassium in the urine, potentially leading to a dangerous lowering of the potassium level in the blood. The 'potassium sparing' diuretics do not have this effect; they should not be given together with potassium supplements or drugs that retain potassium, such as ACE inhibitors, except under strict medical supervision.

Potassium-sparing
Aldactide, Aldactone, Amilco, Amiloride, Berkamil, Diatensec, Dytac, Laractone, Midamor, Spiretic, Spiroctan, Spirolone

Other diuretics
(Some of which are combined with a potassium sparing diuretic or potassium supplements): Aluzine, Aprinox, Arelix, Baycaron, Berkozide, Burinex, Centyl-K, Diamox, Diumide-K, Diurexan, Dryptal, Dyazide, Dytide, Edecrin, Enduron, Esidrex, Frumil, Frusene, Frusid, Hydrenox, Hydrosaluric, Hygroton, Hypertane, Kalspare, Lasikal, Lasilactone, Lasix, Lasoride, Metenix, Metopirone, Moduret 25, Moduretic, Navidrex, Neo-Naclex, Nephril, Normetic, Saluric, Tenavoid, Triamco

OTHER DRUGS USED IN TREATING HEART FAILURE

Heart failure is usually treated with diuretics, but these may be supplemented by two other types of drug—those derived from the ancient drug digitalis (from the foxglove) and the modern ACE inhibitors. These drugs prevent the formation of angiotensin, a substance that causes arteries to constrict. The enzyme involved in this process is called the angiotensin-converting enzyme (ACE); when it is inhibited the blood pressure falls, and the work of the heart is reduced.

ACE inhibitors
Accupro, Acepril, Capoten, Carace, Innovace, Zestril

Digitalis-like drugs
Cedilanid, Lanoxin

7. Angina

In 1786, the English physician William Heberden gave the name 'angina pectoris' to the 'strong and peculiar symptoms' of which some of his patients complained. The word angina has its origins in the Greek *anchein*, which means 'to strangle'. Heberden's account of angina has never been bettered:

They who are afflicted with it, are seized while they are walking (more especially if it be uphill, and soon after eating) with a painful and most disagreeable sensation in the breast, which seems as if it were to extinguish life, if it were to continue; but the moment they stand still, all this uneasiness vanishes.

THE FACTS ABOUT ANGINA

WHAT IS IT?

Angina is a discomfort or pain in, or adjacent to, the chest, which is due to a transiently inadequate supply of blood to the heart muscle. This is not severe enough to cause lasting damage.

WHAT'S IT LIKE?

Classical angina has four typical features:

- its location;
- its character;
- its relationship to exercise and other forms of stress;
- its duration.

The most common place for angina is in the centre of the chest, and it usually seems to be located behind the breastbone (sternum). Very often, however, it is felt in other sites as well, such as the sides of the chest, the lower jaw, and the arms (especially the left) as far as the wrists and hands (Fig. 7.1). Very occasionally, it occurs in the back of the chest or in the upper part of the abdomen. Sometimes, when a person first experiences

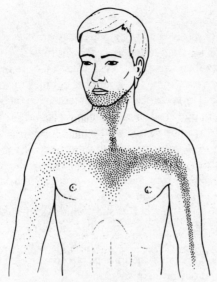

Fig. 7.1. The shaded area indicates common sites for angina.

angina, it is confined to an area, such as the wrist or jaw, which would not suggest the diagnosis were it not provoked by exertion. In most cases, however, it involves the chest to a greater or lesser extent.

Because the heart beat can be felt under the left breast, it is often believed that this is where 'pain in the heart' should be. Although angina may be experienced under the left breast, it is almost never restricted to this area. Indeed, if someone spontaneously complains of 'pain in the heart' one can be confident that the heart is not the cause of the pain.

WHAT DOES IT REALLY FEEL LIKE?

Angina is usually thought of as a pain, and it can be a very severe one, but many sufferers strenuously deny that it is painful, preferring to describe it as a 'discomfort'. The sensation is often likened to a heavy weight on the chest, a strangling or vice-like feeling, or a pressure. Much less often it is described as 'burning' or 'sharp', but in this case the word 'sharp' is being used to mean 'severe' rather than 'like a knife'. In fact, angina is not a stabbing feeling and is often quite a dull sensation. Many patients find it virtually impossible to describe what they feel, and resort to gestures to convey what they are experiencing.

WHAT BRINGS IT ON?

The majority of those who have angina relate it very clearly to exercise; there are some who will initially say that 'it can come on at any time', but later realize that it does not occur when they are resting peacefully. Apart from exercise, there are a number of other important provoking factors, especially anger or fear. Sexual intercourse combining, as it does, exercise and emotion is a common cause. Other factors which aggravate angina include exposure to cold weather and a heavy meal. A particularly likely time for it to occur is when hurrying uphill for a bus, on a cold morning after a large breakfast; in fact, many people find that they get it only when they first go outside in the morning. Quite often, patients will find that they have to stop on several occasions on the way to the bus or train, and will pause in front of shop windows to save them from the embarrassment of being seen to be unable to carry on.

Occasionally, patients experience angina predominantly or exclusively in bed at night. This can sometimes be put down to exciting dreams, but often there is no obvious explanation.

Doctors will always ask a patient with suspected angina how long the discomfort lasts. This is a very difficult question to answer, because it is seldom if ever timed. Most attacks last between one and ten minutes; it is not momentary or over in a matter of seconds, nor is it a persistent ache.

WHAT CAUSES IT, AND WHO GETS IT?

Angina is the result of inadequate blood supply (ischaemia) to the muscle of the heart, although we still do not know exactly why or how the pain is caused. Much the commonest cause is narrowing of the coronary arteries due to atherosclerosis, but there is quite a large number of disorders that may be responsible either alone or in combination with atherosclerosis. Anything that causes the heart muscle to thicken (hypertrophy) may outstrip the ability of the coronary arteries to supply enough blood. Causes of hypertrophy include extreme narrowing of the aortic valve (aortic stenosis), high blood pressure (hypertension), and certain diseases of the heart muscle itself (cardiomyopathies). Angina can also result from coronary artery spasm, severe anaemia, and extremely fast heart rates (as in the disorders of heart rhythm known as paroxysmal tachycardias); these disorders alone seldom cause angina, but commonly aggravate that due to atherosclerosis.

Coronary spasm occurring in otherwise normal arteries is a rare but important cause of angina. It differs from the other types of angina in

being unrelated to exercise or other obvious provoking factors. Indeed, it
is most likely to occur in the early hours of the morning when the victim
is lying quietly in bed. It is sometimes called variant or Prinzmetal's
angina. Much more frequently, angina is caused by quite minor changes
in the activity of the muscles of the coronary arteries, when these occur
in arteries already narrowed by atherosclerosis. Very occasionally,
angina can occur in the absence of any demonstrable abnormality in the
coronary arteries; the term 'syndrome X' has been used to describe this
unexplained disorder.

Because angina is usually due to atherosclerosis, it is mainly encountered in late middle age and in the elderly. The other disease
processes that are responsible for angina can be present at almost any
age; if angina occurs in the young, a very full investigation is called for
to determine the cause.

HOW IS IT DIAGNOSED?

Experienced doctors can usually make a confident diagnosis of angina on
the basis of a carefully taken history alone, but they need to examine the
patient and make a variety of tests to determine its cause and assess its
severity. Listening to the heart with a stethoscope (auscultation), together
with electrocardiography and echocardiography (see Chapter 5) will
usually be sufficient to establish whether one of the less common causes
of angina is responsible, but they will not help in deciding how severely
narrowed the coronary arteries are or how badly the heart is affected.

To make sure that the pain really comes from the heart, it is necessary
to show that it coincides with inadequate blood flow to the heart muscle
(myocardial ischaemia). There are several ways of doing this, of which
the recording of an electrocardiogram (ECG) during exercise on a
treadmill is most popular (see Chapter 5). Unfortunately, this can be
misleading as there may be no ECG changes in the presence of undoubted
angina, and sometimes the depression of the ST segment usually associated with ischaemia occurs in perfectly normal hearts (this feature is
most often seen in young women). An alternative method is nuclear
imaging in which an isotope (e.g. thallium) is used that concentrates in
heart muscle in proportion to the blood flow to that muscle. These tests
help to establish that the heart muscle is poorly supplied with blood, but
they do not provide direct information about the coronary arteries themselves. This can only be done accurately by coronary angiography, a
potentially uncomfortable and (rarely) dangerous investigation seldom
necessary for the diagnosis, but essential if angioplasty or coronary
bypass surgery are being considered (see Chapter 6).

WHAT ELSE COULD THE PAIN BE?

There is a host of conditions that can give rise to pain which can be confused with angina. One of the most important of these is the anxiety state (also sometimes called cardiac neurosis). Sufferers from this complain of sharp, stabbing pains under the left breast or a dull ache in this area. Usually the pain is not related particularly to exercise, and often there is also breathlessness, palpitation, and fatigue. The individual concerned tends to sigh frequently, and to have sweaty but cool hands. A typical example of this was Shirley, a single woman of 36 who had recently lost her father from a heart attack at the age of 61. She complained to her doctor of 'a stabbing pain in her heart', usually when she was in bed, and pointed to a tender spot under her left breast. The doctor noticed that she was sweating profusely and was sighing frequently; putting these various features together, he was confident that she was suffering from an anxiety state but she was not willing to be reassured until she had had an ECG. This was normal and she went away happier although, as explained in Chapter 5, an ECG taken at rest is a poor test for angina.

Disorders of the digestive system can give rise to symptoms that closely resemble angina. This is particularly the case with pain from the oesophagus which is frequently due to the regurgitation of acid from the stomach; it is most likely to occur when lying down (particularly after a large meal), but can sometimes be worsened by exercise.

HOW DANGEROUS IS IT?

To many people, the word angina conveys the idea of early and sudden death. In fact, even in the days before modern treatment, many patients with angina lived for decades, though with varying degrees of disability. Often it comes and goes over many months, sometimes disappearing altogether during the summer and reappearing every winter or when life for some reason becomes more difficult. It has been found that the prognosis in angina is closely related to the number of coronary arteries severely narrowed, so that the outlook is excellent if only one is involved, less good if two are affected, and relatively poor if all three major arteries are implicated. If there is critical narrowing of the left main coronary artery, there is a great risk of death within a few months. The other major determinant of prognosis is the extent of damage to the heart muscle in previous heart attacks.

AMLODIPINE
5 and 10 mg TABLETS

Read all of this leaflet carefully before you start taking this medicine.

- Keep this leaflet. You may need to read it again.
- If you have further questions, please ask your doctor or pharmacist.
- This medicine has been prescribed for you personally and you should not pass it on to others. It may harm them, even if their symptoms are the same as yours.

The name of your medicine is **Amlodipine 5 or 10 mg Tablets.**

- The active ingredient is amlodipine (as besilate).
- Other ingredients are microcrystalline cellulose, calcium hydrogen phosphate, sodium starch glycolate and magnesium stearate.

The Marketing Authorisation holder and company responsible for manufacture: TEVA UK Limited, Eastbourne, BN22 9AG.

1 AMLODIPINE; WHAT IT IS AND WHAT IT'S USED FOR

- Each tablet contains 5 or 10 mg of amlodipine (as besilate). Amlodipine belongs to a group of drugs called calcium-channel blockers. It relieves heart problems by widening blood vessels to allow more blood to flow through. This helps to reduce blood pressure and relieve the strain on the heart muscle.
- The 5 mg tablets are available in pack sizes of 15, 20, 28, 30, 50, 56, 84, 90, 98, 100, 112 and 300 tablets. Not all pack sizes may be marketed.
  The 10 mg tablets are available in pack sizes of 14, 15, 20, 28, 30, 50, 56, 84, 90, 98, 100 and 112 tablets. Not all pack sizes may be marketed.
- Your medicine is used in the treatment of high blood pressure and angina, including the rare form, Prinzmetal's angina.
  Amlodipine does not provide immediate relief of chest pain from angina.

2 BEFORE YOU TAKE AMLODIPINE

Do NOT take Amlodipine if you:
- Are sensitive to amlodipine besilate or any of the other ingredients in your medicine
- Are sensitive to any other calcium channel blockers e.g. nifedipine, felodipine
- Are pregnant, trying to become pregnant, or breast-feeding
- Suffer from unstable angina (excluding Prinzmetal's angina) or aortic stenosis (a narrowing of the main artery leading from the heart)
- Have suffered a collapse of your blood circulation system (cardiogenic shock).

Take special care with Amlodipine if you have:
- Liver problems
- Had a heart attack within the last month
- Suffer from heart failure
- A hypertensive crisis (very high blood pressure).

Pregnancy and breast-feeding:
- Do not take Amlodipine if you are pregnant, trying to become pregnant, or breast-feeding.

3 HOW TO TAKE AMLODIPINE

Your doctor has decided the dose which is suited to you. Always follow your doctor's instructions and those which are on the pharmacy label. If you do not understand these instructions, or you are in any doubt, ask your doctor or pharmacist.

Amlodipine Tablets are for oral use and should be swallowed with a drink of water.

The usual dosage instructions are given below:
Adults (including the elderly)
The starting dose is one 5 mg tablet, once a day. This may be increased to a maximum of 10 mg (two 5 mg tablets or one 10 mg

tablet) once a day.
Children
Not recommended.
If you take more Amlodipine than you should
If you (or someone else) swallow a lot of the tablets all together, or if you think a child has swallowed any of the tablets, go to your nearest hospital casualty department or your doctor immediately. Please take this leaflet, any remaining tablets and the container with you to the hospital or doctor so that they know which tablets were consumed. Overdose may cause redness of the skin and low blood pressure (dizziness and fainting).
If you forget to take Amlodipine
If you forget to take a tablet, take one as soon as you remember, unless it is nearly time to take the next one. Never take two doses together. Take the remaining doses at the correct time.

 4 POSSIBLE SIDE EFFECTS

Like all medicines, Amlodipine can have side effects. If the following happens, stop taking Amlodipine and tell your doctor immediately or go to the casualty department at your nearest hospital:

Difficulty breathing and swelling of the lips, face and neck.

This is a very serious but very rare side effect. You may need urgent medical attention or hospitalisation.

Tell your doctor if you notice any of the symptoms listed below:
Common side effects (affecting fewer than one person in 10 but more than one person in 100):
- Headache
- Water retention causing swelling
- Sleepiness, tiredness
- Abdominal pain, nausea
- Flushing
- Dizziness
- Palpitations.

Uncommon side effects (affecting fewer than one person in 100 but more than one person in 1,000):
- Shortness of breath, fainting
- Indigestion, vomiting, dry mouth, altered bowel habit
- Difficulty sleeping, mood changes
- Impotence, breast enlargement in men

- Problems with urination including an increased need to urinate
- Changes to taste perception
- Low blood pressure
- Blocked or runny nose, sneezing
- Back, muscle or joint pain
- Rash, skin discoloration, increased sweating, itching
- Visual disturbances
- Ringing in the ears
- Loss of sensation, muscle cramps
- Shaking, generally feeling unwell, feeling of weakness
- Hair loss
- Weight increase or decrease
- Chest pain.

Very rare side effects (affecting fewer than one person in 10,000):
- Unusual bleeding or unexplained bruising
- High level of blood sugar
- Inflammation of the blood vessels
- Coughing
- Enlarged gums
- Numbness or tingling in the hands and feet
- Abnormal liver function test results
- Hepatitis
- Jaundice (yellowing of the skin and whites of the eyes)
- Severe, red, itchy skin rash
- Heart attack, irregular heartbeat
- Pancreatitis (inflammation of the pancreas)
- Gastritis (inflammation of the stomach lining) causing abdominal pain.

If you notice any side effects not mentioned in this leaflet, please inform your doctor or pharmacist.

 5 STORING AMLODIPINE

Keep Amlodipine out of the reach and sight of children.
Do not store above 25°C. Store in the original packaging. Keep the blister in the outer carton. Do not use Amlodipine after the expiry date shown on the outer packaging. Do not take these tablets if there are any signs of discoloration or deterioration of the tablets. Return all unused medicines to your pharmacist for safe disposal.
Revised: January 2007

20025220
62137-T

TEVA UK Limited

HOW CAN IT BE TREATED?

If angina is a result of such remediable disorders as anaemia or aortic stenosis, these should be corrected. Atherosclerosis is not so amenable to cure; treatment then has three components: general management, drugs, and interventions such as angioplasty and surgery.

General measures

The diagnosis of angina is one that often produces great anxiety in patients and their relatives, and the good doctor first explains to them that the future is far from gloomy if measures are taken to adjust the way of life appropriately. In many cases, there is no need to take drugs regularly, and in only a minority is surgery or angioplasty required.

Unduly stressful physical and emotional factors should be avoided, but it is wrong to remove all those challenges, which for most of us make life worth living. Many people with responsible jobs thrive on the responsibility and they should not give this up unless it is proving too much for them. Likewise, jobs that involve physical effort are not necessarily harmful. Employers must realize that angina may be only a temporary problem and it is not sufficient reason to terminate employment before treatment has had a fair trial. Close associates of patients with angina should know that the symptom can be readily brought on by anger or frustration, and they should try to avoid circumstances that might provoke this. Exciting programmes on television are, perhaps not surprisingly, a rather frequent cause of angina.

Emotion and the heart

The powerful effect of emotion on the heart is well illustrated by the dramatic case of John Hunter, one of the founders of surgery. Hunter himself said 'My life is at the mercy of any rascal who cares to take it.' His biographer, Home, describes how 'On October the 16th 1793, when in his usual state of health, he went to St. George's Hospital, and meeting with some things which irritated his mind, and not being perfectly master of the circumstances, he withheld his sentiments, in which state of restraint he went into the next room, and turning round to Dr. Robertson, one of the physicians in the hospital, he gave a deep groan and dropt down dead. It is a curious circumstance that, the first attack of these complaints was produced by an affection of the mind, and every future return of any consequence arose from the same cause; and although bodily exercise, or distension of the stomach brought on slighter affections, it still required the mind to be affected to render them severe; and as his mind was irritated by trifles, these produced the most violent effects of the disease. His coachman being beyond his times, or a servant not attending to his directions, brought on the spasms, while a real misfortune produced no effect.'

Exercise

Because angina is usually due to exercise, it is often thought that exercise should be avoided, but that is not so. Lack of exercise leads to deconditioning so that less and less effort is needed to bring on the pain. Angina patients should be encouraged to walk as much as they can, short of producing the pain, but to think carefully when they go out for a walk so they do not find themselves in a situation in which they may have to walk up a steep hill, or into a cold wind on the way home. Angina is most likely to occur on going to work in the morning; plenty of time should, therefore, be allowed for getting to the bus or train. Angina can be brought on by food, but it seldom occurs after meals unless exercise is taken at that time. Certain sports are better avoided, particularly strenuous games such as squash, but those forms of exercise in which individuals can pace themselves, like swimming and cycling, are quite suitable.

Risk factors

Attention must be paid to the risk factors that may have contributed to the development of the disease. This applies especially to cigarette smoking, which aggravates angina in many people but, more importantly, greatly increases the risk of heart attack and death. Raised blood pressure should be detected and, if necessary, treated. It is very unwise for those with angina to be obese, for overweight adds greatly to the work of the heart.

Diet

The importance of a diet that reduces blood cholesterol in patients with angina is a matter upon which medical opinion has in the past been divided. It is probably of less relevance in the elderly, but it should be a routine part of medical management to measure the blood cholesterol in younger patients with angina and to provide dietary advice in accordance with this (see Chapter 4).

Drugs

The three types of drug used in treating or preventing angina—nitrates, beta-blockers, and calcium antagonists—and the ways in which they work are discussed in Chapter 6. The essentials are repeated here.

Choice of drug or combination of drugs

Several factors are taken into account in choosing the anti-anginal drug or combination of drugs for the individual. These include what is thought to be the cause of the angina, the presence of other disorders, such as asthma, diabetes, and hypertension, the history of a heart attack, and the severity of any heart muscle damage. The adverse effects of anti-anginal drugs are largely unpredictable, so that in most cases they can only be discovered once the patient has tried the drug. If new symptoms arise after a drug has been started, a side-effect should always be suspected and the patient should discuss this with the doctor.

Nitrates

The most commonly prescribed drug in angina is glyceryl trinitrate (GTN or nitroglycerin). It is usually taken as a small pill that dissolves while being kept under the tongue. It becomes inactive if swallowed, but it may be chewed. It is absorbed directly from the mouth into the bloodstream and starts working in two to three minutes; its effect lasts for some 30 minutes. Although it abolishes angina quickly, it is most effective when used to prevent an impending attack. It is therefore best to take a tablet when an attack is anticipated—for example, before going out in the morning.

When patients start using it for the first time it may cause quite a severe headache, or lead to dizziness or even a fainting attack. A warning about these possibilities should always be given, and the first tablet should be taken sitting down to see what the result is. These side-effects tend to diminish or disappear with continued use, while it continues to be effective in preventing or relieving angina. There is no limit to the number of tablets that may be taken in a day, but it is unwise to take more than two together. The tablets deteriorate with time; they should preferably be kept in a glass container with no cotton-wool wadding, and should be discarded within six to eight weeks.

An alternative form of glyceryl trinitrate comes as a spray—beware, this is inflammable! The container should not be shaken; two metered doses should be sprayed on or under the tongue, and the mouth closed.

Drugs for angina   1. Nitrates

Administration
Under the tongue ('sublingual')
Aerosol spray
Placed between upper lip and gum ('buccal')
Taken by mouth and swallowed
Self-adhesive patch on the chest wall (absorbed through the skin)

Side-effects
Headache (wears off with continued use)
Flushing
Dizziness
Faintness (sometimes fainting on first use)

Numerous nitrate preparations are used as preventive agents, such as oral isosorbide mononitrate and dinitrate, buccal glyceryl trinitrate tablets (which are left to dissolve after being placed between the upper lip and gum), and self-adhesive patches that deliver the drug through the skin. All these preparations prevent angina if given in sufficient dosage, but they are likely to lose their effect (i.e. tolerance develops) if they are given continuously—a drug-free period is needed in each day. The attempt by manufacturers to provide nitrate cover throughout 24 hours has proved unsuccessful.

Beta-blockers
Beta-blockers dampen the effects of sympathetic nerve activity on the heart, slowing the heart rate and diminishing the force of contraction.

Drugs for angina   2. Beta-blockers
Administration
Oral tablets

Side-effects
Common: fatigue, tiredness, lethargy
Less common: aggravation of asthma or bronchitis, coldness of
    hands and feet, worsening of heart failure, problems with insulin
    control in diabetics, nightmares, depression
Rarely: nausea, diarrhoea, sexual disorders (e.g. impotence), dry
    eyes, rash

They are particularly effective in preventing angina produced by effort or emotion; unlike the nitrates and some calcium antagonists they reduce the risk of a further heart attack in those who have suffered one. On the negative side, they may cause a deterioration in those who already have a severely damaged heart, and cause spasm of the bronchi in those who have a tendency to this (e.g. asthmatics). Furthermore, they make some people feel tired and lethargic, and can cause cold extremities. In spite of these various problems, most patients with angina find treatment with beta-blockers quite acceptable.

Calcium antagonists

Calcium antagonists relax arteries both in the heart and elsewhere. They are of particular value if angina is due to coronary artery spasm, or if angina is of the 'mixed' type, occurring both on exercise and at rest. Although they are often used on their own, it is perhaps commoner to combine them with either nitrates or beta-blockers or both. Some kinds of calcium antagonist (e.g. verapamil and diltiazem) tend to slow the

---

Drugs for angina   3. Calcium antagonists

Administration
Oral tablets
Capsules

Side-effects
Common: flushing, headaches, swollen ankles, constipation
Less common: gastric upsets, dizziness, and fainting

---

heart and are therefore seldom given together with beta-blockers, whereas others (e.g. nifedipine) accelerate the heart and are particularly suitable for this combination. Side-effects include flushing and faintness, headache, gastro-intestinal disorders, swelling of the ankles and, in the case of verapamil, constipation.

Case history—A winter of discontent

Michael is a 70-year-old Yorkshire farmer. He first experienced a heaviness in his chest at the age of 65 when chasing a herd of cattle that had escaped from a field one wintry day. After this he often had what he described as a 'raw' feeling in his chest when he hurried in a cold wind, but the following summer the feeling went away and he thought no more

about it. When the same sensation returned the following November, he
went to see his doctor who gave him glyceryl trinitrate tablets to suck
before he went outside in the cold. At first, these 'blew his head off', but
with continued use he found that he no longer got a headache with
them and they were effective in preventing the angina coming on. A year
or two later, the pain started to come on quite minor exertion. His doctor
then gave him both a beta-blocker (atenolol) and a calcium antagonist
(nifedipine) and he has managed to lead a good life since, although he
doesn't chase animals any longer and mostly stays inside in the winter.

Angioplasty

Angioplasty (see Chapter 6, p. 62) is often effective in relieving angina,
but its success depends on the ability of the operator to pass the balloon
through the narrowed segment of artery and widen the affected vessel at
that point. Initially, angioplasty was used only when a single vessel was
involved close to its origin from the aorta, but as experience has grown
and better equipment become available, multiple narrowings occurring
in several vessels have been tackled. The major drawback of angioplasty
is the risk of totally blocking off a previously open but narrowed vessel
and thereby causing a myocardial infarction. Another unresolved
problem of angioplasty is the liability of the widened vessel to narrow
again during the ensuing six months. Fortunately, in this circumstance,
a second angioplasty is usually successful. Angioplasty is used predominantly when medical treatment has failed to control angina, but only if the
affected artery or arteries are technically suitable for the procedure.

Coronary artery bypass surgery

Coronary bypass surgery (see Chapter 6, p. 65) is very successful in
relieving angina if all the affected vessels are open beyond the sites of
obstruction. The death rate of the operation is low at about 1 to 2 per
cent, provided that the heart muscle has not been extensively damaged
by a previous heart attack. Even when there has been quite a lot of
damage, surgery may be worthwhile—the risk of death from the operation will then be higher, but angina will still be relieved and the risk in
the succeeding years reduced.

The main reason for undertaking surgery is to diminish or abolish
symptoms, but there is good evidence that in certain categories of patient
it substantially improves the prognosis. There is no question that it does
so if the left main coronary artery is severely narrowed; it also seems to
benefit those who have disease affecting all three major arteries if there is

accompanying severe ischaemia, as indicated either by troublesome symptoms, or by a very abnormal exercise test (see p. 45), or by poor function of the heart muscle. Because of this effect on prognosis and because the only way to be sure of the state of the coronary arteries is to undertake coronary arteriography, some cardiologists take the view that everyone with angina should have this investigation. Others feel that one can detect those who would be helped by surgery simply by taking a careful history and by carrying out an exercise test; they confine coronary arteriography to such patients.

Surgery is able to abolish angina in more than half of patients, and substantially reduce it in most of the rest. These benefits are maintained for many years, but atherosclerosis may progress both in the grafts (particularly if veins have been used) and in the patient's natural coronary arteries. This means that angina may recur some time after the operation, and after 10 years it is quite common. Usually, this can be controlled by drugs, but further surgery or angioplasty may be necessary.

Case history—A fisherman's tale

Hamish is a 63-year-old fisherman living in the north of Scotland. In August 1973, he started noticing a tightness in his chest as he walked back home in the evenings, but managed to carry on at work for some months. The pain began to get worse and his doctor gave him glyceryl trinitrate to take before he walked up the hill to his home, but this was not enough, nor were beta-blockers. He was then put off work but he learned about coronary bypass surgery from a television programme. He asked his doctor about this, who was sceptical about its value, but referred him to Edinburgh where he was found, on cardiac catheterization, to have narrowings in all three of his major coronary arteries. After waiting six months for the operation because of a long waiting list, he had coronary bypass surgery. Seventeen years later, he is still working and free of symptoms. The only medicine he takes is aspirin, but he gave up smoking after his operation and is strict about adhering to a diet low in saturated fat. He eats plenty of fish!

UNSTABLE ANGINA

Angina is considered to be unstable if it has started abruptly or has suddenly become much worse for no apparent reason. Often, someone who has had stable angina for months or years finds that over a period of days the discomfort comes on with progressively less effort or even at rest. In most cases, what has happened is that a plaque in a coronary artery has cracked, with platelets and perhaps fibrin becoming attached to its surface, so that artery becomes further narrowed or blocked. Sometimes, coronary artery spasm is superimposed. Fortunately, either spontaneously or with therapy, the process is usually reversed and no serious damage is done. However, in a sizeable proportion of cases, complete obstruction of the artery occurs, with the development of a myocardial infarction. Because of this risk, unstable angina is regarded as a medical emergency, and the patient is usually admitted to a coronary care unit. The symptoms frequently subside with rest and the use of drugs, which are often given in combination. A popular regimen is one of intravenous nitrates with a beta-blocker, but calcium antagonists are often added as well. Either aspirin or heparin, or a combination of the two, are administered in the acute phase, and aspirin is maintained thereafter as it has been found to reduce substantially the risk of a further heart attack in the succeeding years.

If the symptoms do not subside rapidly on medical treatment, coronary angiography is usually undertaken with a view to surgery or angioplasty.

SILENT ISCHAEMIA

Insufficient blood supply (ischaemia) to the heart muscle does not necessarily produce pain, but may cause abnormalities in the tests that are used for angina, such as ST depression on an exercise test or a 24-hour tape recording of the ECG. When such abnormalities are found in the absence of pain, 'silent ischaemia' is said to be present. This can arise in patients who at other times have anginal symptoms but also in individuals with coronary disease who have never had symptoms. It can occur in both stable and unstable angina, and in the convalescent phase after a myocardial infarction. It is still uncertain how important this phenomenon is and whether it needs attention over and above that needed for angina.

8. The heart attack

A heart attack is an acute and potentially serious illness due to coronary heart disease. The term is frequently used to describe sudden and unexplained death as in the typical newspaper announcement:

Mr. Arthur T, the well-known local businessman, died in his sleep on March 4th. It is believed that he died of a heart attack.

It may, however, be quite mild as in:

Mrs. Linda H, of 17 Churchill Avenue, was admitted to hospital last Thursday with a heart attack. The hospital staff said that the attack was mild and she is out of danger.

Most heart attacks of whatever kind result from a sudden event in an already diseased coronary artery, usually a crack in a plaque in the wall of an artery upon which a clot (thrombosis) forms (see p. 13). This leads to partial or complete blockage of the artery; as a result, that part of the heart muscle which it supplies dies (myocardial infarction). The amount of muscle that is affected (and the severity of the heart attack) depends on where the blockage occurs. If the obstruction is close to the origin of the artery from the aorta, a massive amount of muscle may die, and the heart attack may well be fatal, whereas if only a small branch is blocked, the effects are likely to be slight. The extent of damage also depends on the presence or otherwise of collateral vessels—vessels coming from arteries other than the blocked one and supplying blood to the territory threatened by the obstruction. These are not normally present, but develop when there has been an inadequate blood supply over a period of time.

THE FACTS ABOUT A HEART ATTACK

WHAT IS A 'CORONARY'?

This is really an abbreviation of 'coronary thrombosis'. The expression 'coronary' is in widespread use to describe a heart attack, but doctors now seldom describe a heart attack as a coronary thrombosis because clots (thrombi) can form in the coronary arteries without causing a heart attack, and heart attacks are not always due to clots. Doctors usually prefer to use the term 'myocardial infarction' to describe a heart attack, because it is the death of some of the heart muscle that is responsible for most of the problems that arise.

WHAT IS AN ATTACK LIKE AND HOW IS IT RECOGNIZED?

The victim's view of a heart attack is described in detail later in the chapter. In brief, the attack usually starts with a severe pain across the chest, often spreading into the arms (especially the left), and sometimes to the jaw and back. Other symptoms, such as breathlessness, nausea, and faintness, are common and the patient often looks pale and sweaty. A heart attack is usually suspected because of these features, but the diagnosis requires confirmation by one or both of two types of test—the electrocardiogram (ECG) and the measurement of heart enzymes in the blood. The ECG shows electrical changes that reflect injury or death of heart muscle (Fig. 8.1). These occur only over the damaged part of the heart; it is standard to record the ECG from several different sites on the

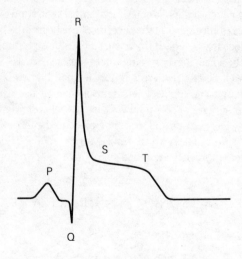

Fig. 8.1. ST elevation in myocardial infarction; compare this ECG with that in Fig. 5.1.

chest so that there is a good chance that it will detect even a small, localized area of damage. The progression of ECG abnormalities over time is characteristic but one cannot be sure from a single recording that a heart attack has taken place, although the features may be highly suggestive.

Heart enzymes are chemical substances contained within the muscle cells that are released into the blood when the cells are damaged by a heart attack. The best known is called creatine kinase; a rise in the blood level of this enzyme is a sensitive marker of a heart attack but it may not rise for some hours after its onset and therefore it, like the ECG, may not be helpful in the immediate diagnosis. A doctor may not, therefore, be able to say definitely whether or not a heart attack has occurred in the early hours after the onset of the pain.

Features of a heart attack

Pain in the centre of the chest, spreading perhaps to both arms (especially the left) and into the lower jaw
It is usually intense and lasts for at least 20 minutes
Often feels like a heavy pressure or is 'vice-like'
Not relieved by aspirin or glyceryl trinitrate

Weakness, occasionally *fainting*

Nausea and sometimes *vomiting*

Shortness of breath

Sweating and *pallor*

WHY ARE HEART ATTACKS DANGEROUS?

Two major types of problem result from the blockage in the artery— electrical and mechanical. Both have their dangers, as do some of the other complications.

Electrical problems
The muscle in the ventricles becomes irritable when it is deprived of blood. Instead of the orderly progression of the heart's electrical current from the atria through to the ventricles (see Chapter 1), parts of the ventricles may start to generate their own electricity. An area may

produce an occasional extra heart beat—usually called a 'ventricular ectopic beat', the word 'ectopic' meaning that it is not coming from the normal place. If these beats successively follow each other regularly at a fast rate (say at a rate of 120 to 200 a minute), this is described as 'ventricular tachycardia'. If this persists for more than a few seconds, it may cause angina or a serious fall in blood pressure.

Ventricular fibrillation

Often, however, the electrical activity in the ventricles becomes completely disorganized, as rapid and chaotic waves of electricity course through the muscle, completely disrupting its regular pumping action and effectively bringing it to a halt. This electrical disturbance, known as 'ventricular fibrillation' (Fig. 8.2), occurs in a substantial percentage of patients with a heart attack and is the commonest cause of death. It usually occurs very soon after the onset, especially in the first hour, but seldom after six hours have elapsed. It does not require a large amount of muscle to be affected to cause ventricular fibrillation and, indeed, most patients seem to be progressing quite well when the cardiac arrest produced by ventricular fibrillation occurs. If the ventricular fibrillation can be corrected promptly, the outcome is usually good, with the patient making a satisfactory recovery.

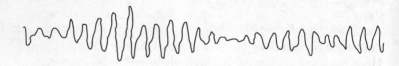

Ventricular fibrillation

Fig. 8.2. Ventricular fibrillation causing complete irregularity of the heart.

Other rhythm disorders

Other less serious electrical disturbances may occur. The atria can also become irritable, and *atrial fibrillation* may develop. This is like ventricular fibrillation in that chaotic electrical activity occurs (Fig. 8.3). Although the atria may beat at a very fast rate, only a minority of these beats can get down to the ventricles through the bundle of His, so that in this disorder, the ventricles tend to beat irregularly at about 120 to 160 a minute. This may create no difficulty if the heart muscle has not

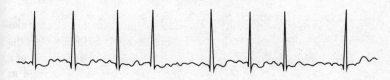

Atrial fibrillation

Fig. 8.3. Atrial fibrillation: Irregular beating of the heart due to atrial fibrillation, irregular undulations replace the P waves.

been extensively damaged, but may impose an intolerable burden if it has, and result in congestion of the lungs. Atrial fibrillation during a heart attack is usually a transient affair, lasting at most a few days.

Another electrical problem arises when the tissue that conducts the current from the atria to the ventricles (the bundle of His) is starved of its blood supply. Often, this leads to some of the impulses not being relayed to the ventricles, so that they beat more slowly than usual, but it is likely to be serious only if there is total interruption of conduction—*complete heart block*. Usually, when the ventricles are completely deprived of electrical stimulation from the atria, they start their own regular activity at about 40 to 60 a minute, but the rate may be less than this or they may fail to generate an impulse at all, in which case the heart stops ('asystole'). *Asystole* can lead rapidly to death, but it is sometimes quite transient, with only a brief period of unconsciousness. The slow heart rate caused by heart block may lead to heart failure or shock (see below). Heart block and asystole can be effectively treated by pacemaking.

Mechanical problems

The pumping (mechanical) activity of the heart depends on the efficient and co-ordinated rhythmic contraction of the muscles of the ventricles. As a result of the heart attack, a portion of the muscle dies and can no longer pump. If something like 40 per cent of the muscle is damaged, a satisfactory circulation cannot be maintained, the blood pressure falls and the state of *shock* exists. This is nearly always fatal.

If the damage is less severe, the heart may not be able to pump out all the blood coming back to it through the veins, and acute heart failure occurs. The term *acute heart failure* is used to describe a condition resulting from the inadequate pumping action of the heart that is associated with congestion of the lungs. It is a potentially serious condition, but advances in treatment in recent years have greatly improved the outlook.

Other complications
Emboli

Emboli are clots that migrate from one part of the body to another through the blood vessels. Some of the most important are those that migrate to the arteries of the lungs (pulmonary emboli) from clots which have formed in the veins in the legs; these are likely to develop in those who lie in bed for a long time. They used to be a common cause of death in heart attack patients when it was fashionable to keep them in bed for weeks, but they have become much less so now that early mobilization is practised. Another important site for emboli is the brain (cerebral emboli); such emboli cause a stroke, the usual consequence of which is paralysis of one side of the body. This affects about 1 per cent of heart attack victims, the source for the emboli usually being in the heart, either from the left atrium (especially if there is atrial fibrillation) or from the area of the left ventricle affected by the muscle damage.

Rupture

Death of muscle may soften it and make it prone to rupture. Blood under pressure in the left ventricle may burrow through the outer wall of the heart, so that blood accumulates in the pericardium which surrounds it. This usually leads quickly to death. Rupture may also affect the septum that separates the two ventricles, so that blood pours through from the high-pressure left ventricle to the low-pressure right ventricle. This usually leads to death within hours or days but may be treatable by surgery. Finally, the muscles that support the mitral valve may rupture and lead to a severe leak back through the valve. This, too, is often fatal but minor degrees of rupture may not be serious.

Pericarditis

The damage to the heart may extend to the outer surface of the muscle and may then irritate the covering layer of pericardium. The inflamed pericardium may give rise to a central chest pain on the second to fourth day after the onset, and this may suggest that there has been a further heart attack. It differs from the pain of the heart attack in being sharper and being made worse by breathing in. It also can give rise to a scratchy noise that the doctor can hear with a stethoscope. It is not a serious complication and usually settles down within a few hours.

Aneurysm

The muscle in the affected area tends to become thinned and replaced by a thin layer of scar. This may bulge outwards each time the remaining normal muscle contracts; the paradoxically moving, bulging area is known as an aneurysm. This wastes much of the effort expended by the normal muscle and can lead to heart failure in the months following the attack; surgical removal of the aneurysm with repair of the wall of the heart is often successful.

WHAT IS THE RISK OF DYING FROM A HEART ATTACK?

A heart attack victim is at high risk of a cardiac arrest in the first hour or so after its onset but this risk falls quickly thereafter. Once six hours have elapsed, patients who by then look and feel well usually progress very satisfactorily. On the other hand, those who are breathless, have troublesome disturbances of heart rhythm, or who have a low blood pressure, are in greater danger of further complications. Twenty-five years ago, 25 to 30 per cent of patients admitted to hospital with a heart attack died; today the figure is 5 to 10 per cent. The risk of death is very dependent on the age of the patient. The death rate in hospital of those under 50 years is probably less than 3 per cent, and not much greater in those between 50 and 60, whereas those over 75 are at a much higher risk.

This great improvement in outlook in recent years has resulted from intensive observation and treatment in the first day or two, with the prompt correction of cardiac arrest and the prevention of major muscle damage by the use of such drugs as those that dissolve the clot.

WHAT ARE THE LONG-TERM EFFECTS OF A HEART ATTACK?

Most survivors of a heart attack recover well and only a small portion of the muscle of the heart is replaced by a scar. Such people may be completely free of problems and are able to return to a normal life. Others have sustained more severe damage, and may experience breathlessness and other symptoms because the heart has not enough muscle to pump efficiently. In between are a group of patients in whom the damage is moderate, but who have angina because they still have one or more narrowed coronary arteries. There is, therefore, a wide range of degrees of recovery after a heart attack, and advice and treatment must be individualized as there are few rules that apply to all patients.

IS THERE A RISK OF A FURTHER HEART ATTACK?

Anyone who has had a heart attack is susceptible to another, but the risk of a recurrence diminishes with time, and can be substantially reduced by appropriate measures (such as not smoking, and by the use of aspirin and beta-blockers). In fact, a further heart attack is most likely to occur in the days immediately after the first and tends to follow a recurrence of angina. If there is no recurrence by one year after the first attack, the risk reduces progressively thereafter so that after some years there is little more risk than in those who have never had an attack.

THE PATIENT'S AND RELATIVES' VIEW OF A HEART ATTACK

WHAT DOES IT FEEL LIKE?

Pain

The outstanding feature of most heart attacks is the pain. It is often extremely intense, and far worse than anything the patient has ever experienced. It is usually in the centre of the chest, and is described variously as vice-like, a heavy pressure, squeezing, or tight. The pain often spreads to the lower jaw, and the arms (especially the left), and may go through to the back. Some patients suffer only mild pain and they may think it is due to indigestion, for which it is often mistaken.

Occasionally there is no pain at all, and it is only when an ECG is taken some time later that it is discovered that a heart attack has taken place.

The pain may start abruptly, but more often it increases progressively to its peak, or comes and goes over a period of minutes or hours. Unlike the pain of angina, it is not provoked by effort or exertion, nor is it relieved by glyceryl trinitrate tablets—it usually requires a very potent drug, such as morphine or heroin, to control it.

Sometimes the pain of a heart attack is the first experience the patient has had of heart pain, but more often it is preceded by a progressive increase in the severity of pre-existing angina or the development of angina for the first time in the preceding days (unstable angina; p. 85).

Other symptoms

Although for most patients, the pain is the main complaint, other symptoms may occur and indeed may be more distressing than the pain. Some patients feel very weak or faint during the early hours of the attack and may actually lose consciousness briefly. Breathlessness, sweating, and nausea (and less often vomiting) also occur—though nausea and vomiting are also often due to the pain-relieving drugs.

These symptoms usually subside within one-half to three hours, either spontaneously or as a result of pain-relieving drugs, but can last much longer. Many patients feel surprisingly well once the pain has gone, and may find it difficult to believe that they can have experienced a heart attack. Others may develop the pain of pericarditis or feel 'washed out' over the next few days, but a small proportion of patients feel and are seriously ill with heart failure or shock; they may feel exhausted or become breathless.

Anxiety

It is natural to feel anxious when you have a severe pain, and even more so if you think that you are having a heart attack. It is not surprising, therefore, that anxiety is usual at this time, and can be made worse by the atmosphere of panic that a heart attack may engender amongst family and colleagues, by the drama of an ambulance journey, and by admission to an unfamiliar hospital environment. Most patients are now admitted to a Coronary (or Cardiac) Care Unit (CCU); the staff in these units are highly professional and can usually provide the reassurance that quickly calms the nerves. Sometimes, however, the presence of a mass of electronic apparatus can appear alarming if it is thought to imply that the patient must be critically ill. It is essential for the staff to explain that this equipment is part of the routine.

Anxiety usually diminishes rapidly once the patient becomes accustomed to the environment, but it may surface again at the time of transfer from the CCU to an ordinary ward. The patient, having adapted to life in the CCU, may feel less protected away from the intensive observation and from the close relationships that develop with the nurses there.

Anxiety may occur for similar reasons on going home, but it is liable to give way to depression. Only when the patient returns to familiar surroundings may the full significance of the heart attack be appreciated. For many people it may be the first time that they have been brought face to face with their mortality. A man may have to face the fact that he cannot return to a physically demanding job. For women, the transition back home may be particularly difficult. They may have similar employment worries as men, but they may also be expected by their families to return immediately to their domestic duties of ironing, housework, and cooking. For others, a completely different situation may obtain—the mother who for a lifetime has provided all the comforts of a home finds that her family can cope perfectly well without her and she loses her sense of purpose. Resolving these various domestic situations demands understanding on the part of all concerned.

WHY ME AND WHY NOW?

Some patients with heart attacks undoubtedly conform to the stereotype of the stressed, overworking, overweight, heavy smoking, middle-aged man, but most are unremarkable in any way. Such people cannot understand why they should be the subject of such misfortune and nor can their doctor. While it is true that most heart attack subjects have one or more of the risk factors, and the majority smoke, it is seldom that there is an obvious explanation for an attack occurring when it did. Every doctor has seen a few cases which have clearly been the consequence of some dramatic event, such as that of the 40-year-old miner who developed severe chest pain when he was on all fours protecting a colleague beneath him after the roof of the mine fell in. Relatives, especially spouses, like to have an explanation of the attack and are apt to attribute it to stress at work or domestic conflicts, but only rarely do claims of this kind withstand critical examination. It is also often said that the patient has been unusually tired prior to the attack, but this tiredness may well have been an early feature of the heart problem rather than a sign of stress.

HOW DOES A HEART ATTACK APPEAR TO RELATIVES AND FRIENDS?

In many instances, it is very obvious to the bystander that the patient is seriously ill. He or she is in severe pain, and is pale and sweaty. Often, unlike in angina, patients may be restless, trying to walk around or to find a more comfortable position. They may retch or vomit, or become breathless, or may fall unconscious either due to a simple faint or to a cardiac arrest. In milder cases, the victim may not look ill, and appears no different from someone with indigestion. Once the pain has subsided, the patient looks normal or tired.

During the next few days, there is little change in the appearance, although he or she may seem tense or depressed. Once home, he or she may seem weak and lacking in energy. Very often, with the depression that occurs at this time, the patient may be withdrawn or irritable for no apparent reason. The family must not become upset by outbursts of temper, and should not respond with anger.

WHAT CAN RELATIVES AND FRIENDS DO IF THEY SUSPECT A HEART ATTACK?

At the time

A heart attack should be suspected in anyone who develops a severe pain in the centre of the chest, and this should be assumed to be the diagnosis, unless there is good reason to make an alternative one. It may be difficult in someone who already has angina to know whether a chest pain is a heart attack or simply a rather worse than usual episode of angina. The pain of a heart attack is usually both more severe and long-lasting; angina seldom lasts for more than 15 minutes, and will subside with rest and the use of glyceryl trinitrate under the tongue. Furthermore, in angina it is unusual to be pale or sweaty, or to be nauseated or vomit.

Quick action is essential in a heart attack, and the patient must be brought under skilled medical or paramedical care as soon as possible. Whether to call for an ambulance or the general practitioner (GP) depends upon local circumstances. If the patient's GP is known to belong to an immediate care scheme (e.g. BASICS), or if one is really in doubt as to the problem, it is best to call him or her. Otherwise, it is best to call for an ambulance, and to explain that this is a suspected heart attack.

Patients should be placed in a position in which they are comfortable—usually slightly propped up. However, if they look pale and shocked they should lie flat but if breathless they may want to sit up straight.

If the patient should become unconscious, it is vital to decide whether this is due to a simple faint or to a cardiac arrest. In a faint, a pulse can be felt in the neck and recovery is quick when the subject is lain flat. A cardiac arrest should be diagnosed in anyone who becomes unconscious if no pulse can be felt in the neck. One should immediately start basic life support.

In hospital

Once the patient is in hospital, the role of relatives and friends is different —it is mainly to keep up the morale of all concerned. Good visiting in hospital is an art. It used to be the case that visiting times were very limited; then it was easy to decide how long to stay. With more prolonged or even free visiting, it is difficult to know how long to spend with the patient. Much as most patients like to have visitors, it can be very tiring, especially if there are many on the same day (some of whom may need to be kept apart from one another!). Conversation should be based on the reasonable assumption that the patient will make an excellent recovery. However, if the patient wants to discuss serious problems, such as the return to work or the making of a will, these should not be avoided. It is right for close relatives to learn from the medical or nursing staff the true condition of the patient, but it is as well to remember that forecasting the outcome of a heart attack is only marginally better than weather forecasting—unexpected hurricanes sometimes do happen.

At home

The problems for the relatives really begin when the patient comes home; it is not easy to be a good husband or wife to a heart attack victim. One has to steer a middle course between 'wrapping the patient in cotton wool' and letting them get back to a full life too quickly. In deciding how to cope with this situation, it is essential to know:

- how severe the heart attack has been;
- how much exercise was allowed before hospital discharge, and how much is recommended over the next month;
- what medicines have been prescribed and how they should be taken;
- what untoward features should act as a warning that further medical attention is necessary.

Smoking must be absolutely discouraged; diet needs to be prudent rather than extreme, unless special instructions have been given. Usually, the patient will have been walking about the ward or up a flight of stairs before discharge from hospital, and can gradually increase this day by day after returning home, going outside if the weather is not wet or cold. The family and friends must be prepared for the anxiety or depression that may develop (particularly if these have been a problem in the past), and for the irritability that is common at this time. All this requires patience and understanding. Happily, most patients make an excellent physical and psychological recovery, and many consider the heart attack as giving them a new lease of life.

WHAT TREATMENT IS GIVEN TO A PATIENT WITH A HEART ATTACK?

At the time

Heart attacks most commonly start in the home, and if this is the case the first medical person on the scene is usually the GP. If he or she thinks that a heart attack is likely, morphine or heroin is usually given to relieve the pain. Then, the decision has to be made as to whether the patient should be transferred to hospital. In favour of going to hospital is the high risk of cardiac arrest and other complications in the first few hours, which can best be combated by the facilities offered by a hospital. Against it are the possibility of a long ambulance journey, the anxiety that leaving one's home and entering an unfamiliar environment may engender, and the fact that after a few hours have elapsed the risk of serious problems is small in the patient who looks and feels well. Ambulance workers today are mostly well-trained and equipped to look after heart attack patients and are able to deal with any emergencies that may arise.

In hospital

The ambulance usually delivers the patient to the Accident and Emergency (Casualty) Department of a hospital. This tends to be very busy, and it may take some time for the doctors to assess the situation, take an ECG and decide whether to send the patient to the CCU.

The CCU is an area specifically designed to take care of patients who have heart attacks. Its purpose is to ensure that those who are suspected of having had a heart attack are under close observation by specially trained nurses and doctors. Frequently, patients are accommodated in single or double rooms with glass walls so that they can be seen readily while not being exposed to the noise so typical of hospital wards. An essential component of coronary care is the use of electrocardiographic monitoring. This involves attaching two or three electrodes to the chest wall, which are connected by wires to oscilloscopes (visual display units) located both at a central station and at the bedside. By this means, the rhythm of the heart is continuously displayed, so that any disturbance can be treated immediately.

It is usual for a needle to be inserted into a vein on the back of the hand or in the forearm, and left in place there. This enables the staff to withdraw blood for tests and give drugs without the need for further needling. It may be necessary, however, to insert other needles or tubes. A catheter may be passed via a vein in the arm, groin region or neck to record pressures in the right side of the heart or pulmonary artery; this may be done if there is heart failure or shock, because a knowledge of the level of pressure in the heart is valuable in deciding how much of a drug may be necessary to keep up the blood pressure or relieve congestion in the lungs. A special type of catheter with an inflatable balloon on its tip (known as a Swan–Ganz catheter) is commonly used for this purpose; it floats with the blood stream through the right side of the heart to the pulmonary artery. Another type of catheter is one with an electrode in it; this may be passed to the right ventricle and used for electrically stimulating (pacing) the heart when it is beating too slowly due to heart block.

Drugs

Drugs (see Chapter 6) which are usually administered during the heart attack include pain-relieving opioids (e.g. morphine and heroin), aspirin, and thrombolytic drugs (to dissolve the clot). No more drugs may be necessary, but beta-blockers and nitrates (by mouth or intravenously) and heparin (either intravenously or subcutaneously) may be given. If the patient is breathless or the lungs are congested, digitalis (digoxin) or a diuretic may be used and, if there is low blood pressure, drugs such as dopamine or dobutamine may be infused through a vein.

When can I get up and when can I leave the Unit?

The speed of mobilization depends on the speed of recovery and the practice of the individual Unit. Most patients can sit out of bed on the second or third day, and discharge from the CCU to the ward also usually takes place about this time. If, however, the blood pressure has been low, if there has been recurrent pain or breathlessness, or if there has been a disturbance of the rhythm of the heart, both mobilization and transfer may be delayed.

What happens between discharge from the CCU and discharge from hospital?

This time is spent in getting strength back in the legs, making sure the heart attack is really over, and deciding on what investigations and drugs are needed before convalescence. An opportunity is now taken to start rehabilitation, and the patient should receive counselling on the way of life he or she should follow in the future. Physiotherapists will usually supervise exercises, either for the individual or in groups, and other health professionals such as rehabilitation nurses and occupational therapists also may be involved.

The medical staff will attempt to assess the state of the heart with repeated physical examinations, with chest X-rays, and ECGs. In many hospitals, a short exercise test will be carried out about a week after admission (see Chapter 5). This will usually be done on a treadmill, walking at a speed of about 2 miles per hour for 8 minutes. It tests both the heart and general fitness. If a patient is unable to complete this test, or develops angina or major ECG changes, it may be decided to undertake other tests which may include coronary angiography. If the exercise test is passed with flying colours, this is very reassuring and usually implies that the outlook is excellent.

On discharge

Patients usually go home on the seventh to tenth day but this depends on the home circumstances and on the speed of recovery. By the time of discharge, the patient is usually walking comfortably about the ward and, perhaps, up and down one flight of stairs.

Most patients leave hospital on two or more drugs. The use of beta-blockers and aspirin is almost routine, as both in their different ways reduce the risk of further heart attacks. However, beta-blockers may not be given if there has been heart failure, or if the outlook seems to be so good without them that they are not thought to be necessary. Other drugs may include diuretics, digitalis, and ACE inhibitors if there has been heart failure, and anti-arrhythmic drugs, if there is considered to be a risk of serious rhythm disturbances.

Poor recovery

A few patients make a slow recovery and may need a prolonged period in hospital. This may be because of continuing angina. If this is so, consideration will be given to performing angioplasty or bypass surgery at an early stage. However, most of these patients will make a satisfactory recovery with anti-anginal drugs and may well require the use of calcium antagonists and long-acting nitrates.

Another major problem is persistent heart failure. This is usually the result of extensive damage to the heart muscle. While the damage may be irreversible, drug treatment is usually effective in controlling the breathlessness and fatigue that are the main symptoms. Sometimes the heart failure is due to an aneurysm, which can be treated by surgery.

Case history—Troubled times at the Foreign Office

Ernest Bevin was British Foreign Secretary from 1945 to 1951, but throughout this period, and even before it, he suffered from heart trouble. His symptoms seem to have begun as early as 1937, at the age of 56, but the first serious problem was attacks of unconsciousness attributed to heart block in 1945. He recovered from these, but went on to have several heart attacks, recurrent angina, and severe breathlessness until his death in 1951. Today, his heart block could have been effectively controlled with a pacemaker, and undoubtedly with the several types of drug now available he would have suffered much less from chest pain and breathlessness, and would probably have lived several more years.

9. Rehabilitation after a heart attack

The purpose of rehabilitation is to restore the individual to a full and enjoyable life. To do this, it is essential that their whole personality and physical well-being is taken into account. Everyone who has had a heart attack needs advice about such things as diet, smoking, exercise, and work. Many benefit from an organized programme, started in hospital and continued in a rehabilitation centre.

THE WAYS AND MEANS OF REHABILITATION

DIET AND CHOLESTEROL

Patients who are overweight should try to get their weight down to the acceptable range for their height (see pages 33–4), so that the heart is not having to support an unnecessarily heavy load.

Most patients who have had a heart attack have a cholesterol level higher than ideal and should adopt the dietary principles described in Chapter 4. Cholesterol-lowering drugs may be given to patients who have high blood cholesterols that do not respond to diet.

ALCOHOL

Moderate alcohol drinking is neither bad for the heart, nor is it good. Many patients find that a glass or two of wine a day is comforting, but larger amounts are to be discouraged.

SMOKING

Smoking is an important cause of heart attacks, and is even more dangerous in those who have had one already. Smoking must therefore be completely stopped, and close associates should avoid subjecting the patient to passive smoking. Although cigars and pipes are probably less risky, it is wiser not to smoke at all.

EXERCISE

All patients should be advised before leaving hospital about the amount of exercise they can take when they go home. Generally speaking, patients will have been walking around the ward and perhaps up a few stairs before they are discharged; if they have been managing this easily in hospital this can be taken as the starting point at home. Gradually, over the next week or two, the amount of walking may be increased and this can be supplemented by the use of a stationary bicycle. Within a few days, the patient can go for walks outside if the weather is not cold or windy, and can attempt gentle hills after a few more days. Within two to three weeks, it should be possible to walk a mile or two, and this can be progressively increased over the next four to six weeks. Progress will be slower if exercise produces angina or breathlessness. If these symptoms are present, medical advice is necessary; they will usually diminish with treatment and exercise can then be increased.

In the longer term, certain forms of exercise, such as squash and weight-lifting, should be permanently avoided, but less energetic forms of sport such as tennis, golf, and badminton can usually be enjoyed as can swimming (in warm water) and cycling. Although some patients after heart attacks get back to more vigorous sports such as skiing and even marathon running, these should not be attempted until a gradual build-up has shown that no adverse effects result from lesser forms of effort; even then medical advice should be obtained.

SEXUAL INTERCOURSE

One of the greatest worries that many patients have after a heart attack is about the return to intercourse. Both patient and partner may be concerned that it will impose too great a strain on the heart. The physical effort used in intercourse is much the same as that of walking up two flights of stairs, but the strain on the heart may be much greater if intercourse is very vigorous or if it is intensely emotional. Return to gentle sexual activity is usually quite safe some four weeks after the attack, provided recovery has been good.

Sexual difficulties may arise at this time. There may be a loss of libido and males may find they are impotent. These problems most often result from anxiety or depression and resolve when these factors diminish. They can also be due to drugs such as beta-blockers and diuretics.

Doctors and nurses often fail to mention this subject spontaneously;

patients and their partners should not hesitate to ask questions about their worries.

STRESS

Although in this book little emphasis has been placed on stress as a *cause* of heart disease, it can be a very important factor in determining the success of rehabilitation. It is essential that patients, relatives, colleagues, and health professionals all appreciate this. It is also necessary to recognize the strain that a heart attack imposes on those close to the patient— fear of death of a loved one, worries about the future with regard to occupation or finance, and feelings of guilt that somehow they may have contributed to the attack.

Domestic problems that have existed before the heart attack may be greatly aggravated by it, although where there are basically sound family relationships, these may be reinforced by the re-evaluation that takes place because of the life-threatening event.

Previous stress in the workplace may discourage return to work; discussion with colleagues or employers may help to resolve this.

Relaxation exercises, yoga, and similar techniques may be valuable in allowing the individual to 'unwind'. Rehabilitation programmes are often most helpful in overcoming stress-related problems.

ANXIETY AND DEPRESSION

Some degree of anxiety is normal after a heart attack, but it can be quite disproportionate and then requires treatment. Concern about a further heart attack is natural, but reassurance that this becomes increasingly unlikely with the passage of time, particularly if the patient takes the appropriate steps to prevent it, will usually lead to resolution of these fears.

Depression tends to start after return home, although it can be a problem in hospital too. Often it is only when patients are faced with everyday domestic life that the implications of their illness truly 'come home'. Depression is not always easy to recognize because it may manifest itself as fatigue, tiredness, irritability, and easy loss of temper. It is obviously aggravated by concern over future health and the ability to return to work, as well as by the anxiety of the partner. It may vary greatly from day to day, the patient one day feeling that he or she is back to normal and the next day feeling exhausted and dispirited.

If patients and those close to them realize what the problem is and its temporary nature, it can be overcome by understanding. The patient's complaints should not be laughed off; they merit serious discussion. The family in particular must not be discouraged if the patient's failure to be reassured seems irrational. In the course of time, a more optimistic attitude will usually return.

RETURN TO WORK

Those who have been in work before their heart attack are usually keen to get back to their old job, although a significant proportion take the opportunity to go into retirement, which they might have been planning in any case.

From the purely physical point of view, most patients are fit for light work, perhaps part-time, in about eight weeks. More strenuous occupations may be resumed at about 12 weeks, but it is usually not possible to go back to heavy work. However, after discussion with employers and colleagues it is often possible to modify the work previously done in order to avoid the heaviest jobs. Today, few jobs are heavy and a commoner problem is the stress involved in the work, and the travelling to and fro. Again, understanding employers will reduce the workload and not exert too much pressure in the weeks following resumption of work, but patients are often concerned that promotion will be compromised or the job actually downgraded. Employers should realize that those who have recovered from a heart attack, like others who have been disabled, may be more conscientious than ever before. The Disablement Resettlement Officer should be involved, if appropriate, soon after the heart attack, if it seems probable that there will be difficulty in re-employment.

INSURANCE

It is as well for patients who have had heart attacks to inform their life insurance company. Some companies will permit further or new life insurance when there has been a good recovery from a heart attack—an insurance broker will provide details. Medical insurance should be taken out for travel abroad.

DRIVING

Heart attacks seldom cause road accidents, but they can do so and it is natural that there should be restrictions on drivers with heart disease. This is particularly the case in the first month after an attack.

Ordinary licence holders may return to driving after one month, if they are free of symptoms; those who have angina when they drive should not do so. Those who are disabled after a heart attack should inform the Driving and Vehicle Licence Centre in Swansea. In all cases, it is wise to inform the driver's insurance company as the heart attack may affect the cover provided.

Those who drive passenger-carrying or large goods vehicles (previously designated PSV or HGV licence holders) are usually precluded from doing so subsequently.

FLYING

Flying as a passenger in a modern commercial aircraft imposes little risk, even for a patient with quite serious heart disease. The cabin is pressurized to an altitude of 5000 to 6000 feet, and oxygen is available should this prove necessary. Some aircraft even carry defibrillators. It is, therefore, not unreasonable for a patient who has made a good recovery from a heart attack to fly two or three weeks after the attack.

Nonetheless, it is usually wise to defer journeys by air somewhat longer, not so much because of the dangers of flying but because of all the problems and delays that can arise in airports. It is important that the airline is informed of a patient who has recently had a heart attack as the process of boarding and disembarking can be made much easier by the use of porters, wheelchairs, or buggies.

REHABILITATION PROGRAMMES

Formal rehabilitation programmes have been developed on a large scale in the United States and continental Europe. Less than half of British hospitals have them although they are becoming more common.

There are two essential components to such programmes—counselling and physical retraining. Both should start before hospital discharge, but the formal out-patient programme usually commences some four weeks after discharge and may continue for up to six months. Patients attend two or three times a week, with a structured programme of exercises suitable for each individual. At these sessions, the patient's personal problems are discussed, attempts are made to deal with stress, and relaxation exercises are taught.

Patients usually find rehabilitation worthwhile; it succeeds in convincing most that they can return to a full life in the near future.

Certainly, such programmes are likely to hasten the return to work—unless attendance at the classes actually impedes this. However, there are many patients who return quickly to full activity without such help; these are likely to be those with a stable home background and a supportive family.

SELF-HELP GROUPS

Those who have recovered from a heart attack often find it helpful and reassuring to discuss their problems with others who have been through similar experiences. When they have overcome their own problems they may like to provide advice and encouragement to those who have yet to do so. Self-help groups composed of such people can be very supportive and may supply a focus of interest to those who would otherwise be lonely or lacking in purpose. They may arrange communal events (such as lectures on relevant subjects, and visits to the theatre or seaside), and also become involved in fund-raising for the local hospital or other charitable causes. A list of such groups is available from the Chest, Heart and Stroke Association (see Appendix B).

Case histories—Presidential coronaries

In 1952, Dwight Eisenhower was elected President of the United States at the age of 62. Three years later, when he was playing a round of much-loved golf, he was interrupted by several phone calls, some of which proved to be false alarms. After having a lunch consisting of a large hamburger and raw onion, he started another round but this was again interrupted and he lost his temper. About this time, he developed 'an uneasiness' in the stomach that he attributed to 'my injudicious luncheon menu'. That evening, he developed the classical features of a heart attack.

Two months later, in November 1955, he returned to work, but apparently in the succeeding few weeks he was thought by his close associates to be depressed, though subsequently he himself denied this. Nonetheless, by February of 1956 he was considered by his cardiologist, the famous Dr. Paul Dudley White, to be able to carry on an active life satisfactorily for a further five to ten years. In fact, he was re-elected President later that year and completed his second four years in office in 1960. He eventually died at the age of 79 in 1969.

In 1955, 47-year-old Lyndon Baines Johnson was a hard-working senator, who smoked some 60 cigarettes a day and was 2 to 3 stones overweight. When driving in the Virginia countryside (only a couple of days after having had a routine ECG reported as normal), he developed nausea, a sense of constriction in his chest, and a heaviness in the arms. He was found to have sustained a heart attack from which he made an excellent recovery. Eight years later, he became President of the United States after the assassination of President Kennedy, and he was re-elected by a huge majority in 1964.

These case histories illustrate how full a recovery can be made from a heart attack. One can imagine no more stressful job than that of these two American Presidents, one holding office during one of the worst periods of the Cold War, and the other facing intense unpopularity at the time of deteriorating fortunes in Vietnam.

Two other observations are worth making from these stories—in the case of Eisenhower, the mistaking of a heart attack as indigestion and in the case of Johnson, the fact that a normal ECG is no guarantee of a normal heart.

Appendix A: Glossary

Aneurysm. A thinned area of the wall of the heart or aorta which bulges outwards each time the heart contracts.

Angina pectoris. Discomfort in the chest and adjacent areas due to inadequate blood supply to the heart muscle.

Angiogram. A moving X-ray picture of the heart and blood vessels, obtained after the injection into the blood of a fluid which is opaque to X-rays.

Angioplasty. A procedure in which a tiny balloon on the end of a cardiac catheter (q.v.) is used to widen a narrowed coronary artery.

Anticoagulant. A drug that reduces the clotting capacity of the blood.

Aorta. The main artery (q.v.) conducting blood from the heart.

Artery. A blood vessel that carries oxygen-rich blood.

Asystole. Complete cessation of the heart's electrical activity.

Atheroma. Deposits of fatty material and cholesterol in blood vessels.

Atherosclerosis. Atheroma with fibrous tissue and sometimes calcium deposits.

Atrial fibrillation. Very rapid and chaotic electrical activity in the atria.

Atrium. One of the two (left and right) receiving chambers of the heart.

Auscultation. Listening to the heart sounds, usually with a stethoscope.

Bundle of His. A narrow bundle of fibres that are normally the only route by which electricity can pass from the atria to the ventricles.

Capillaries. Very small blood vessels interposed between the arteries and veins, through the walls of which oxygen, carbon dioxide, and other substances pass to and from the tissues beyond.

Cardiac. Pertaining to the heart.

Cardiac arrest. Complete cessation of the heart beat.

Cardiomyopathy. A disorder of heart muscle; usually the cause is unknown.

Cardiopulmonary resuscitation. The techniques of treating arrest of the heart and/or respiration by artificial respiration and cardiac compression.

Catheter, cardiac. A long, narrow tube which, when passed through the veins or arteries, is used for measuring pressures in the heart, or injecting substances opaque to X-ray for outlining the heart and blood vessels.

Cholesterol. A chemical substance which is in many foods and also found in all cells in the body. Most of the cholesterol in the body is manufactured in the liver. An important constituent of atheroma.

Collateral arteries (vessels). New vessels that grow from an adjacent territory into an area inadequately supplied with blood because of a narrowed artery.

Coronary arteries. The arteries that supply the heart muscle with blood; they arise from the aorta.

Coronary (or Cardiac) Care Unit. A Unit designed for patients with heart attacks and other heart problems in which there are specially trained medical and nursing staff, and the equipment necessary for treating cardiac emergencies.

CPR. Cardio-pulmonary resuscitation.

Defibrillator. An instrument for delivering an electric shock, used to terminate fibrillation (q.v.).

Diabetes mellitus. A disease in which there is excess sugar in the blood, associated with the passage of sugar in the urine.

Diastole. The period during which the heart is resting between beats.

Diuretic. A drug which increases the amount of urine passed.

ECG. Electrocardiogram (q.v.).

Echocardiogram. The record obtained from ultrasound waves reflected from the various structures of the heart.

Electrocardiogram. A recording of the electrical signals from the heart obtained from electrodes positioned on the chest wall and limbs.

Embolism. The migration through the blood stream of a clot from one part of the body to another.

Endocardium. The inner lining of the heart.

Epidemiology. The study of diseases as they affect populations.

Fibrillation. Fast, irregular electrical activity of the atria or ventricles.

Fibrin. Protein fibres which form the basis of clots.

Fibrinogen. The precursor of fibrin normally present in the blood.

Gamma camera. A camera that detects the gamma rays emitted by radioisotopes (q.v.).

HDL. High density lipoprotein (q.v.).

Heart block. Partial or complete interruption of the conduction of electricity from the atria to the ventricles.

Heart failure. A condition in which the pumping action of the heart is inadequate. It can result in the accumulation of fluid in the body and congestion of the lungs.

High density lipoprotein. A complex of fat and protein that tends to remove cholesterol from the tissues. Sometimes described as the 'good' form of cholesterol.

Hypercholesterolaemia. Excessive cholesterol in the blood.

Hypertension. High blood pressure.

Hypertrophy. Excessive thickening of the heart muscle.

Infarction. Death of cells.

Ischaemia. Inadequate blood supply.

LDL. Low density lipoprotein.

Lipid. Fat.

Lipoprotein. A complex of fat and protein.

Low density lipoprotein. A complex of fat and protein which is associated with an increased risk of coronary disease.

Monocyte. A type of white cell involved in the development of atheroma.

Monounsaturated fat. A form of unsaturated fat of which olive oil is the best-known example.

Myocardial infarction. The death of a segment of heart muscle.

Myocardium. The heart muscle.

Nuclear imaging. A technique in which a very small dose of radio-isotope is injected into the blood and its activity in the heart is detected by a gamma camera (q.v.) positioned over the chest.

Oesophagus. The gullet.

Oestrogen. One of the female hormones.

Pacemaker. A part of the heart that can generate its own electrical activity. An artificial pacemaker is an electrical device for stimulating the heart.

Pericardium. The membrane that surrounds the heart.

Plaque. A deposit of atheroma.

Plasma. The fluid of the blood (i.e. without the blood cells).

Plasmin. A substance that dissolves fibrin clots.

Plasminogen. The inactive precursor of plasmin in the blood.

Plasminogen activator. Substance that converts plasminogen to plasmin.

Platelets. Small blood cells that clump together to form clots.

Polyunsaturated fat. A form of unsaturated fat that appears to protect against coronary disease—found in many vegetable oils.

Progestogen. One of the female hormones.

Prothrombin. Precursor of thrombin in the blood.

Radioisotope. A radioactive chemical. Used in very small quantities in nuclear imaging.

Saturated fat. A form of fat that when consumed increases the blood cholesterol; found mainly in meat and dairy products.

Sinus node. The normal pacemaker of the heart, situated in the right atrium.

Sphygmomanometer. An instrument for measuring blood pressure.

Systole. The period during which the heart is contracting.

Technetium. A radioisotope used for labelling blood cells.

Thallium. A radioisotope that concentrates in heart muscle.

Thrombin. Substance which acts on fibrinogen to form fibrin.

Thrombolysis. The dissolving of a clot.

Thrombosis. The process of clotting.

Thrombus. Clot.

Ventricle. One of the two main pumping chambers of the heart.

Ventricular fibrillation. Fibrillation of the ventricles.

Ventricular septal defect. A defect in the septum (wall) separating the two ventricles.

Appendix B: Helpful organizations

Action on Smoking and Health (ASH), 5–11 Mortimer Street, London W1N 7RH. (071) 637 9843
Provides advice and information on giving up smoking.

British Heart Foundation, 14 Fitzhardinge Street, London W1H 4DH. (071) 935 0185
Provides free leaflets on many aspects of heart disease. Several videos are available, including two on heart surgery, one on cardiopulmonary resuscitation ('Don't just stand there!'), and one entitled 'Lower your cholesterol', which is on sale in retail outlets.

Chest Heart and Stroke Association, CHSA House, Whitecross Street, London EC1Y 8JJ. (071) 490 7999
CHSA (Scotland), 65 Castle Street, Edinburgh EH2 3LT. (031) 225 6963
Information, advice, and leaflets on rehabilitation; video on rehabilitation after a heart attack.

Coronary Prevention Group, 102 Gloucester Place, London W1H 3DA. (071) 935 2889
Leaflets on the prevention of coronary disease, and rehabilitation after a heart attack; video on rehabilitation after a heart attack.

Family Heart Association, Wesley House, 7 High Street, Kidlington, Oxon. OX5 2DH. (0867) 570292
Information and advice for those with an inherited tendency to coronary disease.

Health Education Authority, Hamilton House, Mabledon Place, London WC1H 9TX. (071) 383 3833
Responsible for the 'Look after Your Heart' programme and provides general information and leaflets.

Inter Heart (Mike Preston), 60 Barry Road, Netherhall, Leicester LE5 1FB. (0533) 431194
Information on self-help groups.

Take Heart (George Morland, National Chairman), 55 Flaxpiece Road, Claycross, Chesterfield. (0246) 862462 evenings only.
For people who have had heart attacks. Counselling and social activities.

Zipper Clubs (Fred Roach, Executive Chairman), 'Belmont', 30 Perne Road, Cambridge CB1 3RT. (0223) 247431
For patients before and after heart surgery.

Appendix C: Useful cookbooks

The New BBC Diet Book by Barry Lynch, BBC Books, London 1990

Eating for a Healthy Heart. Good Housekeeping. Headline Book Publishing plc, London 1988

Food should be Fun (free from the British Heart Foundation, 14 Fitzhardinge Street, London W1H 4DH, but donations are appreciated)

The Light-Hearted Cookbook by Anne Lindsay, Grub Street, London 1991

Index

120 Index

hyperlipidaemia 25, 29
  familial 25
hypertension 6, 23, 37

infarction, myocardial 7, 13, 87-102
insurance 106, 107
ischaemia,
  myocardial 7, 74
  silent 86

LDL 9, 20, 113
lipoprotein 9, 10, 20, 113
low density lipoprotein 9, 20, 113
lysis 9

monitoring 99
monocyte 8
monounsaturated fat 10, 113
myocardial infarction 7, 13, 87

nitrates 52,71, 81, 100
nuclear imaging 48, 77

oesophagus 78
oestrogen 25, 42
overweight 19, 22, 32

pacemaker
  artificial 100
  cardiac 4
pain
  angina 75
  heart attack 94
pericardium 1, 113
pericarditis 92
personality: Type A 24
plaque 7, 10, 13
  fissure (rupture) of 12
plasma 7, 113
plasmin 9, 113
plasminogen 9, 113
plasminogen activator 9, 113
platelets 8, 113
  aspirin and 56
polyunsaturated fat 10, 21, 113
progestogen 25, 42

prothrombin 8, 114
pulmonary embolism 92

rehabilitation 100, 103-109
risk factors 19, 28, 80
rupture of heart 15, 92

salt 22, 31
saturated fat 10, 21, 30, 114
screening 40
self-help groups 108
sex hormones 25, 42
sexual intercourse 70, 104
  after heart attack
shock 15, 91
silent ischaemia 86
sinus node 4, 114
smoking 22, 36, 71, 98, 103
social class 24
spasm, coronary 13, 76, 114
streptokinase 58, 100
stress 24, 40, 105
stroke 92
sugar 22, 31
systole 6

tape-recording of ECG 47
thallium 48, 77, 114
thrombin 8, 114
thrombolysis 58, 114
thrombolytic drugs 58, 100
thrombosis 8, 114
thrombus 8, 54, 114
triglycerides 10, 20

unstable angina 85

ventricle 1, 114
ventricular fibrillation 14, 60, 90, 97, 114
ventricular septal defect 15, 114
vitamins 22

weight tables
  men 33
  women 34
work after heart attack 106